The Surgical Atlas of

Airway and Facial Trauma

Comprehensive Surgical Atlases in Otolaryngology and Head and Neck Surgery

Editor-in-Chief

K. J. Lee, M.D., F.A.C.S.

Director, Ear Research and Educational Center
Chairman, Education and Research Committee
Coordinator, Laser Surgery Center
President, Hospital of St. Raphael Medical Staff
Chairman, Medical Board
Hospital of St. Raphael
New Haven, Connecticut
Attending, Hospital of St. Raphael, Yale–New Haven Hospital, and Milford Hospital
New Haven and Milford, Connecticut
Consultant, Backus Hospital and Windham Community Hospital
Norwich and Willimantic, Connecticut
Assistant Clinical Professor, Department of Surgery
Yale University School of Medicine
New Haven, Connecticut

The Surgical Atlas of Otology and Neuro-otology
Eiji Yanagisawa, M.D., F.A.C.S., and Gale Gardner, M.D., F.A.C.S.

The Atlas of Head and Neck Surgery
Bruce W. Jafek, M.D., F.A.C.S., and Clarence T. Sasaki, M.D., F.A.C.S.

The Atlas of Aesthetic Facial Surgery
Douglas D. Dedo, M.D., F.A.C.S.

The Surgical Atlas of Airway and Facial Trauma
Robert H. Miller, M.D., F.A.C.S.

The Atlas of Cleft Lip and Cleft Palate Surgery
Howard W. Smith, M.D., D.M.D., F.A.C.S.

Foreword

In the five volumes in this series, the editors, contributors, and I have attempted to illustrate succinctly the current acceptable techniques in otolaryngology and head and neck surgery. When possible and appropriate, we have included alternative techniques for comparison.

I am greatly indebted to the editorial staff of Grune & Stratton, Inc., for their support and patience. I also thank the volume editors, contributors, and illustrators for enduring my numerous phone calls and letters. As usual, my wife and family have been most supportive.

In recognition of our teachers, the volume editors have dedicated these texts to their mentors.

K. J. Lee, M.D., F.A.C.S.
Editor-in-Chief

The Surgical Atlas of
Airway and Facial Trauma

Robert H. Miller, M.D., F.A.C.S.

Associate Professor, Department of Otorhinolaryngology and Communicative Sciences
Baylor College of Medicine
Houston, Texas

Illustrated by

Patrick McDonnell
David M. Bolinsky

G&S

GRUNE & STRATTON
A Subsidiary of Harcourt Brace Jovanovich, Publishers
New York London Paris San Diego San Francisco São Paulo Sydney Tokyo Toronto

Library of Congress Cataloging in Publication Data

Miller, Robert H. (Robert Harold), 1947–
The surgical atlas of airway and facial trauma.

(Comprehensive surgical atlases in otolaryngology and head and neck surgery)
Bibliography
Includes index.
1. Airway (Medicine)—Wounds and injuries—Atlases.
2. Respiratory organs—Wounds and injuries—Atlases.
3. Face—Wounds and injuries—Atlases. I. McDonnell, Patrick. II. Bolinsky, David M. III. Title.
IV. Series. [DNLM: 1. Facial injuries—Surgery—Atlases. 2. Larynx—Injuries—Atlases. 3. Trachea—Injuries—Atlases. WE 17 M649a]
RF51.M5 1983 617'.51 83-12725
ISBN 0-8089-1594-0

Grune & Stratton, Inc.
111 Fifth Avenue
New York, New York 10003

Distributed in the United Kingdom by
Grune & Stratton, Inc. (London) Ltd.
24/28 Oval Road, London NW 1

Library of Congress Catalog Number 83-12725
International Standard Book Number 0-8089-1594-0
Printed in the United States of America

To

Bobby R. Alford, M.D.

Olga Keith Wiess Professor and Chairman, Department of Otorhinolaryngology and Communicative Sciences
Baylor College of Medicine
Houston, Texas

Paul H. Ward, M.D.

Professor of Surgery and Chief, Division of Head and Neck Surgery
UCLA School of Medicine
Los Angeles, California

The two men who have most influenced my career in otolaryngology.

Contents

Preface

Otolaryngologists have been involved in the care of trauma patients for many years, and as the scope of otolaryngology and head and neck surgery expands, the otolaryngologist must be prepared to care for a variety of injuries. Trauma surgery is somewhat unique in that although injuries may fall into broad categories, each injury is sufficiently different to challenge the surgeon's skill. Trauma surgeons must have the ingenuity to modify their knowledge to each situation: it may be that a "standard" reduction of a facial fracture can be achieved, or it may be necessary to apply two or three different techniques with modifications to achieve a satisfactory result. Furthermore, there is no one "right" way to manage any injury. Only by having the knowledge of a wide variety of techniques can head and neck trauma surgeons provide optimal care for their patients. It is hoped that the procedures outlined in this volume, along with the ingenuity and judgment of the surgeon, will lead to the achievement of this goal.

I would like to acknowledge the people who have helped in the preparation of this volume. I am deeply indebted to Patrick McDonnell, who did all of the art except for that in Chapter 8 and without whom this book would not have been possible. His artistic ability as well as his advice is greatly appreciated. Dr. David Shelton did an outstanding job of outlining the basics of a myriad of techniques that are available for the management of mandibular fractures. I also would like to thank Dr. K. J. Lee for inviting me to participate in the series of *Comprehensive Surgical Atlases in Otolaryngology and Head and Neck Surgery* and for his contribution to this volume.

Contributors

David W. Shelton, D.M.D. *Professor, Department of Surgery, Dental Branch*
University of Texas Health Science Center at Houston
Houston, Texas

1
General Procedures

PHYSICAL EXAMINATION

This section is concerned with specific findings for which the physician must search in a patient who has suffered head and neck trauma. This examination is not in place of but rather in addition to a complete examination of the patient.

The postauricular area is examined for ecchymosis (Figure 1-1). This is Battle's sign and is suggestive of a temporal bone or basilar skull fracture. A hemotympanum is also suggestive of a temporal bone fracture.

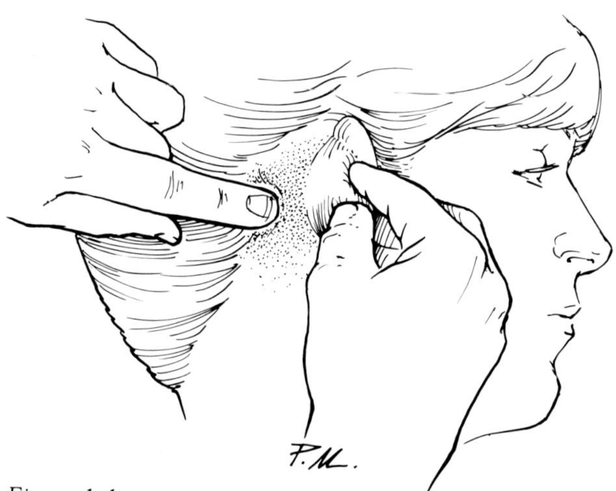

Figure 1-1

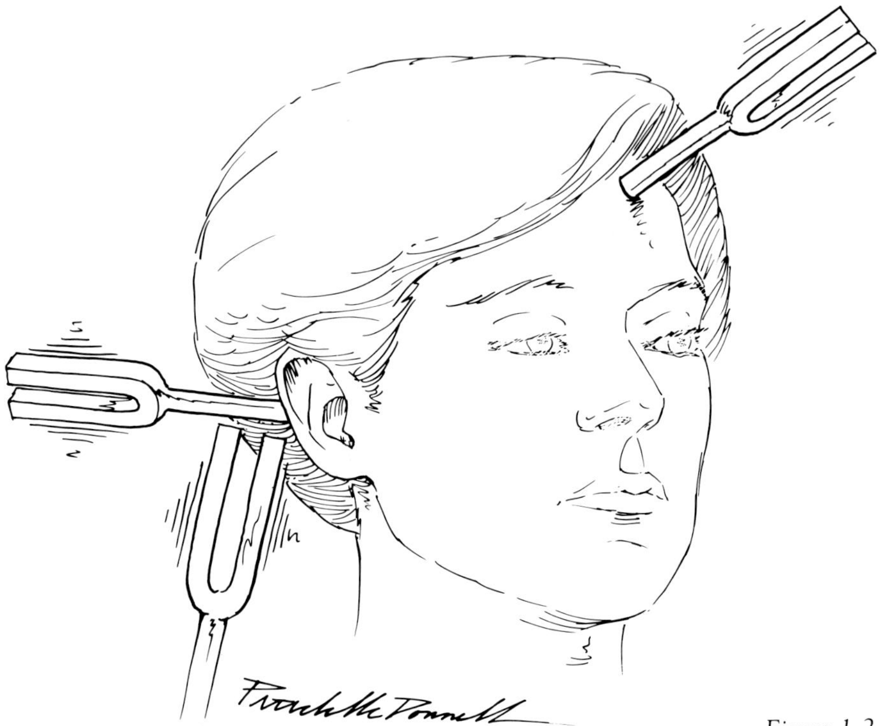

Figure 1-2

The tuning fork examination, including the Weber and Rinne tests, is used to ascertain the status of the patient's hearing (Figure 1-2).

A very important part of the initial ear examination is to assess facial nerve function, since the therapy for facial paralysis may be modified by whether the onset of the paralysis is immediate or delayed (Figure 1-3).

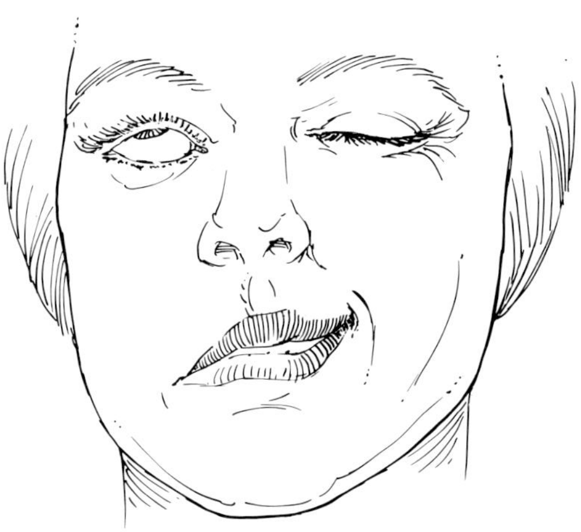

Figure 1-3

Visual acuity and the movement of the globe in all four quadrants is assessed (Figure 1-4). The size of the pupils and their reaction to light must be noted. Fundoscopic examination is also essential to rule out an intraocular injury.

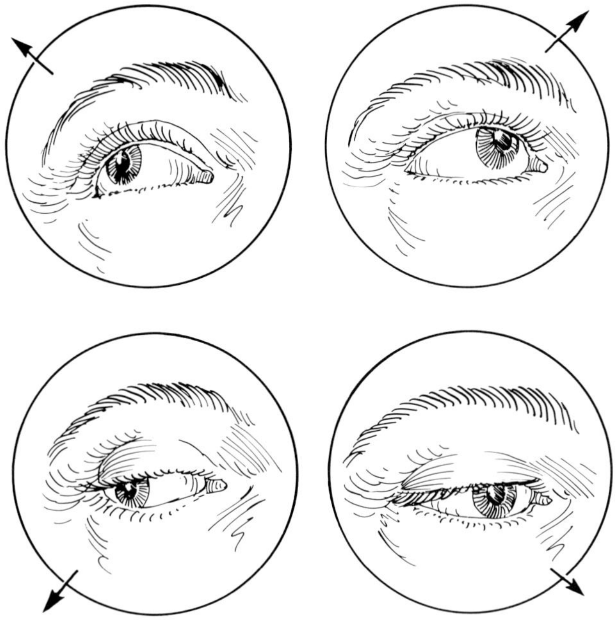

Figure 1-4

All aspects of the orbital rim are palpated to look for tenderness and a palpable step-off (Figure 1-5).

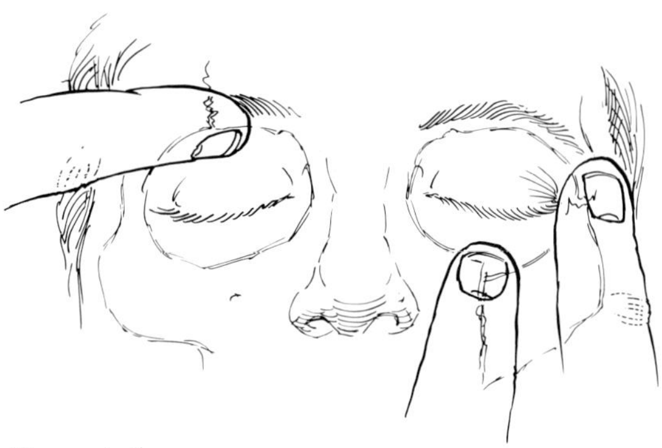

Figure 1-5

The nose is palpated to look for tenderness and deformity (Figure 1-6).

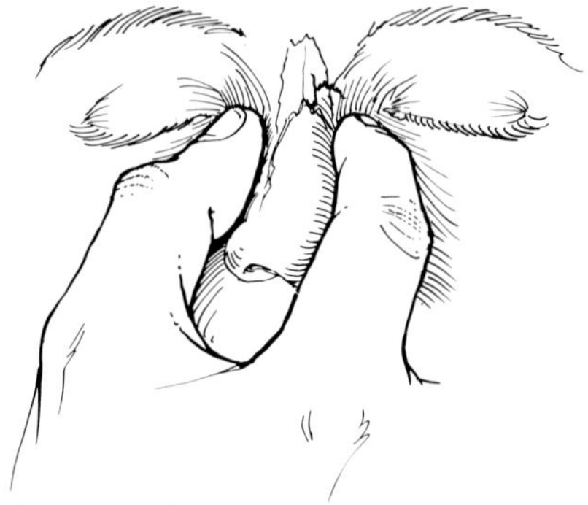

Figure 1-6

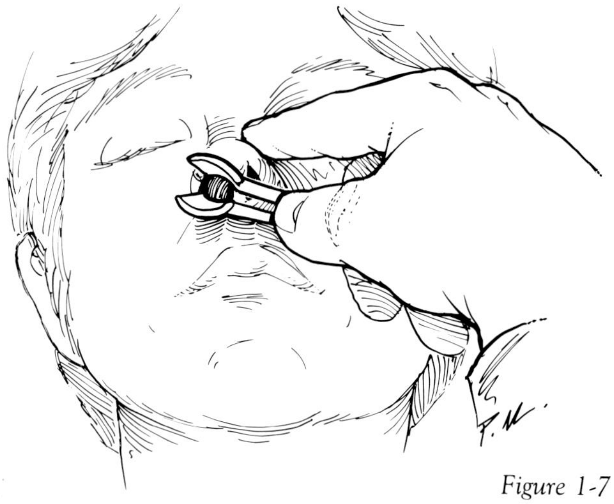

Figure 1-7

The internal aspects of the nose are examined with particular attention to bleeding, cerebrospinal fluid rhinorrhea, and septal hematoma (Figure 1-7).

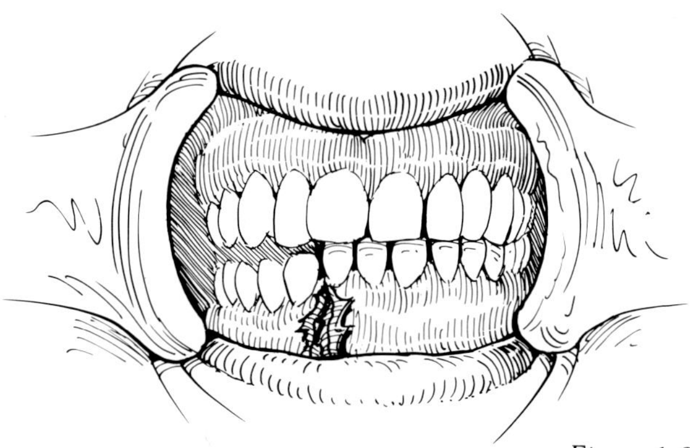

Figure 1-8

The patient's occlusion is carefully examined, and the patient is asked if the occlusion feels normal (Figure 1-8). Intraoral lacerations may indicate an underlying fracture.

The mandible is palpated both extraorally and intraorally (Figure 1-9).

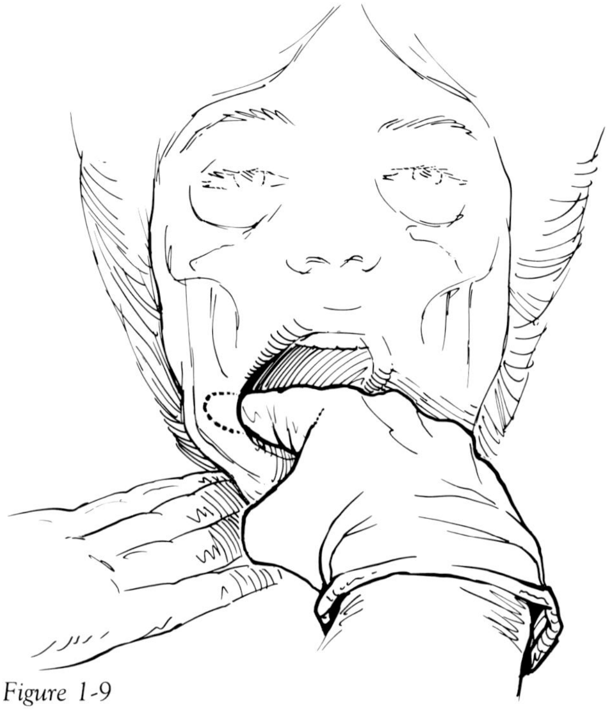

Figure 1-9

The mandible is manipulated bimanually to check for tenderness and mobility (Figure 1-10).

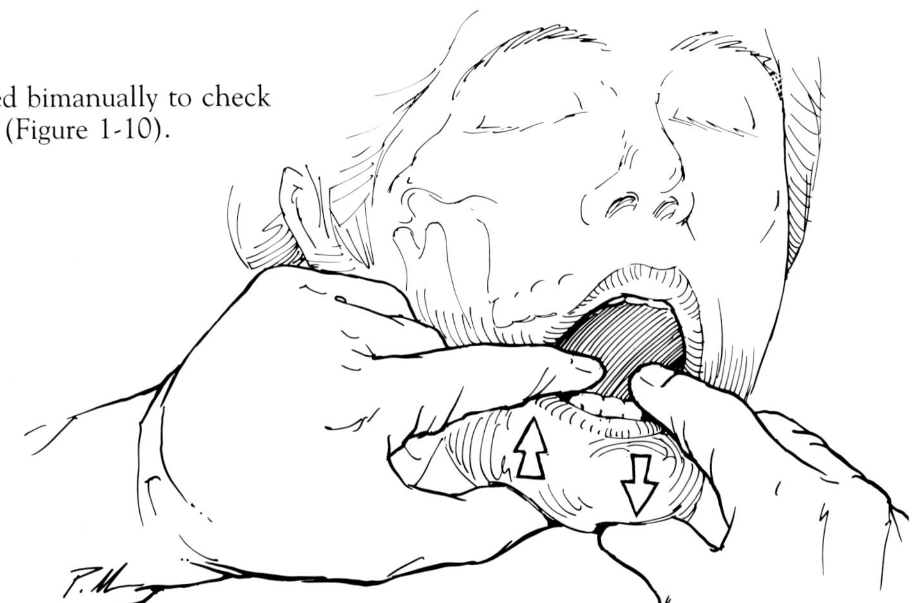

Figure 1-10

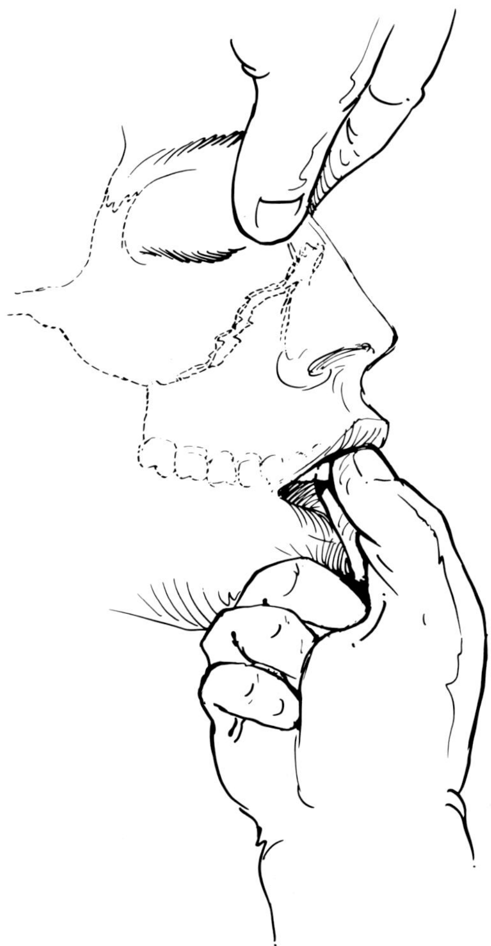

Figure 1-11

The maxilla is tested for mobility (Figure 1-11).

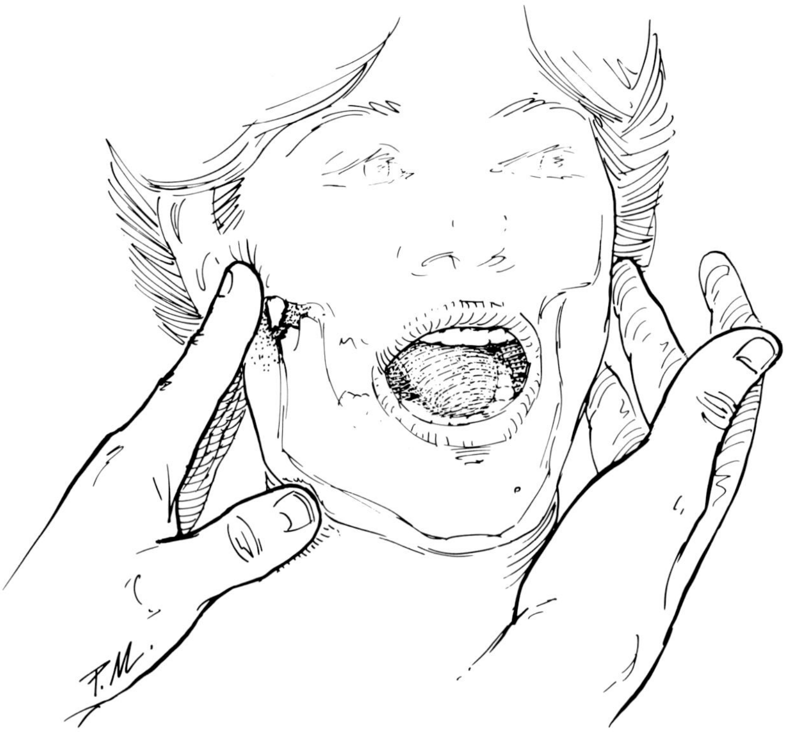

Figure 1-12

The condyles are palpated to assess mobility when the patient opens the mouth (Figure 1-12). A difference in movement on one side may suggest mandibular injury.

A tongue blade is inserted between the teeth on one side (Figure 1-13). If a mandibular fracture is present, pain will accompany movement of the fragments when the patient attempts to achieve occlusion.

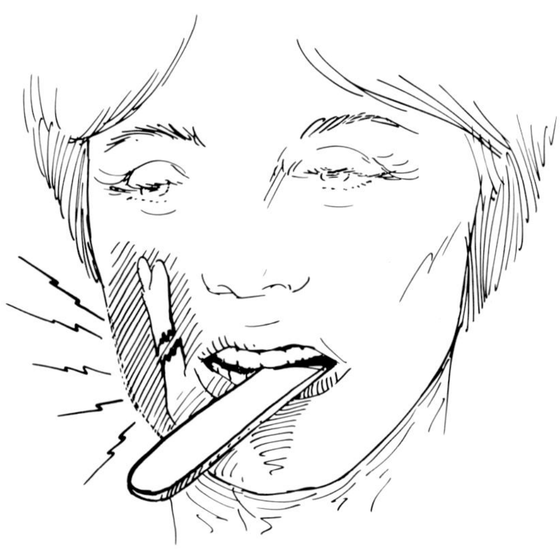

Figure 1-13

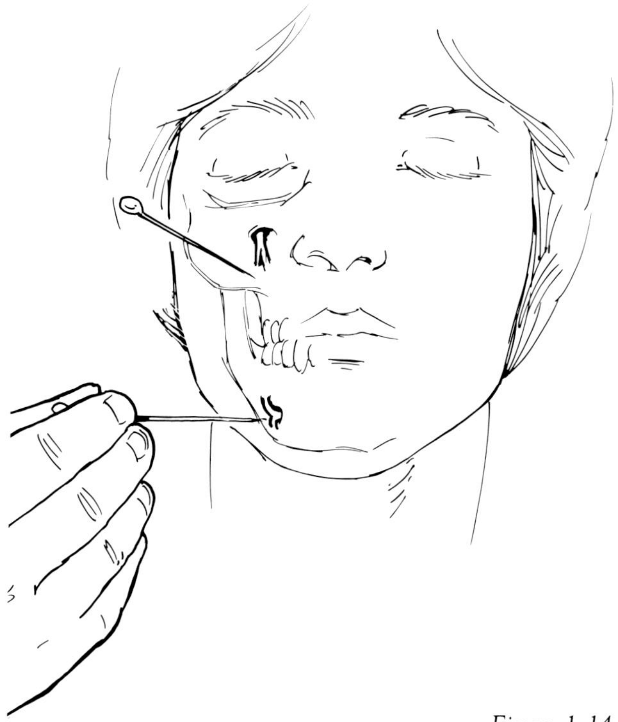

Figure 1-14

Sensation over the cheek, upper lip, and mental area are examined (Figure 1-14). Numbness in these areas may suggest injury of the infraorbital or mental nerves.

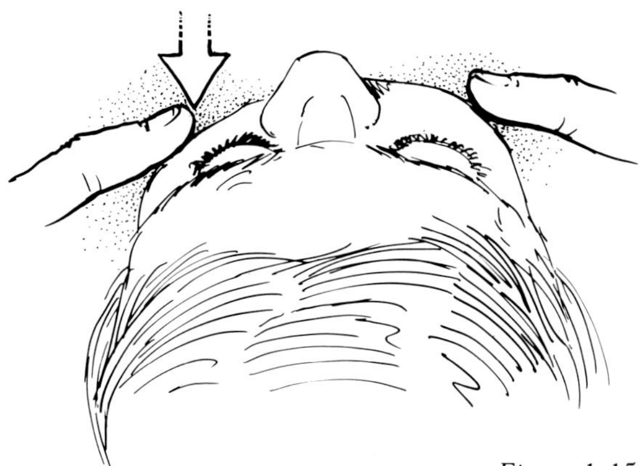

Figure 1-15

By standing behind the patient and looking over the patient's head, one can compare the malar areas (Figure 1-15). Acute swelling may make an initial judgment of depression difficult.

Indirect laryngoscopy is performed to assess not only evidence of mucosal lacerations but also vocal cord function (Figure 1-16).

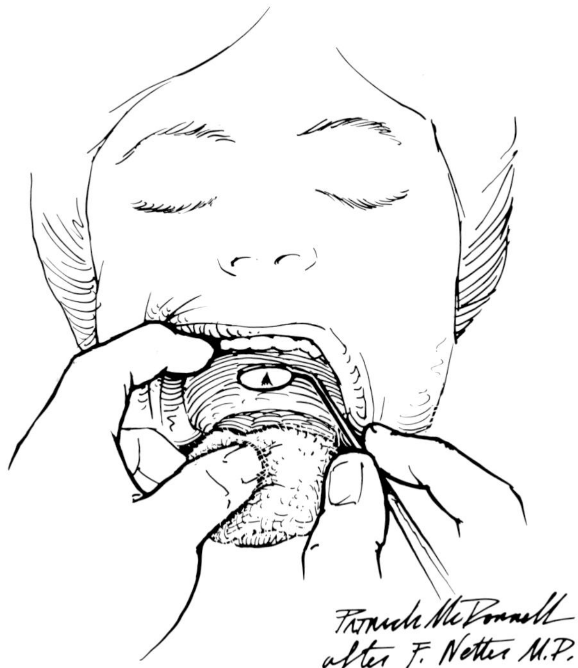

Figure 1-16

The laryngeal cartilages are palpated carefully to look for crepitus, tenderness, deformity, and subcutaneous emphysema (Figure 1-17).

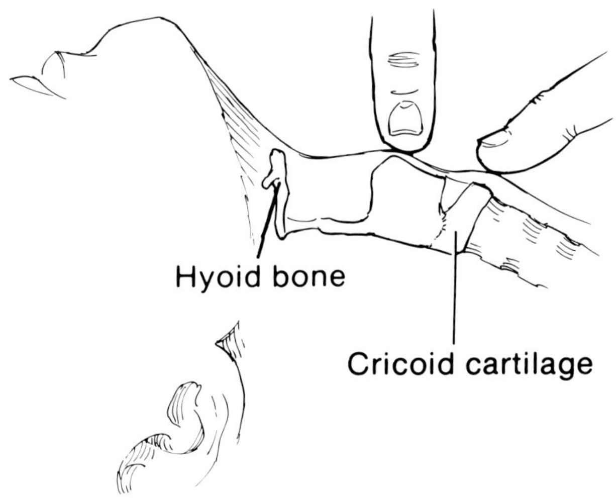

Figure 1-17

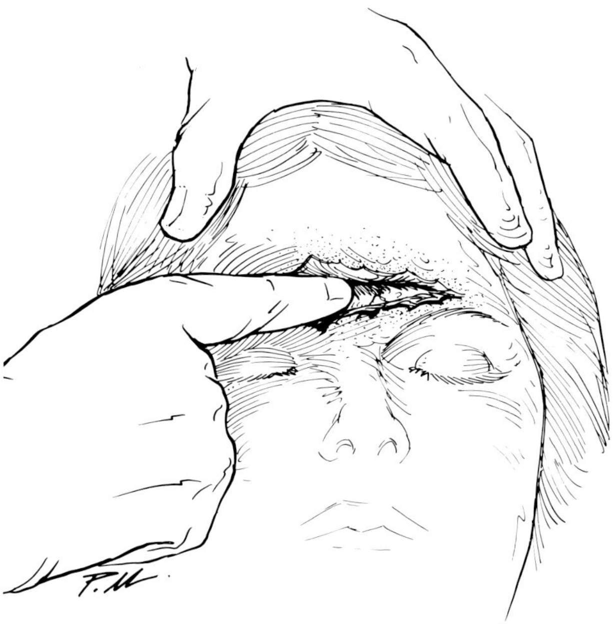

Figure 1-18

The area over the frontal sinuses is palpated (Figure 1-18). If a laceration exists, the bone can be examined directly.

TRACHEOTOMY

Tracheotomy may be lifesaving in the acute situation such as a laryngeal fracture. It may be useful as a way of delivering anesthesia or maintaining an airway in a patient with massive facial swelling. Whenever possible, it should be performed in the operating room under controlled conditions.

An area 1–2 cm below the cricoid prominence is infiltrated with approximately 5 ml 1% lidocaine with epinephrine 1:100,000 prior to preparing the patient (Figure 1-19).

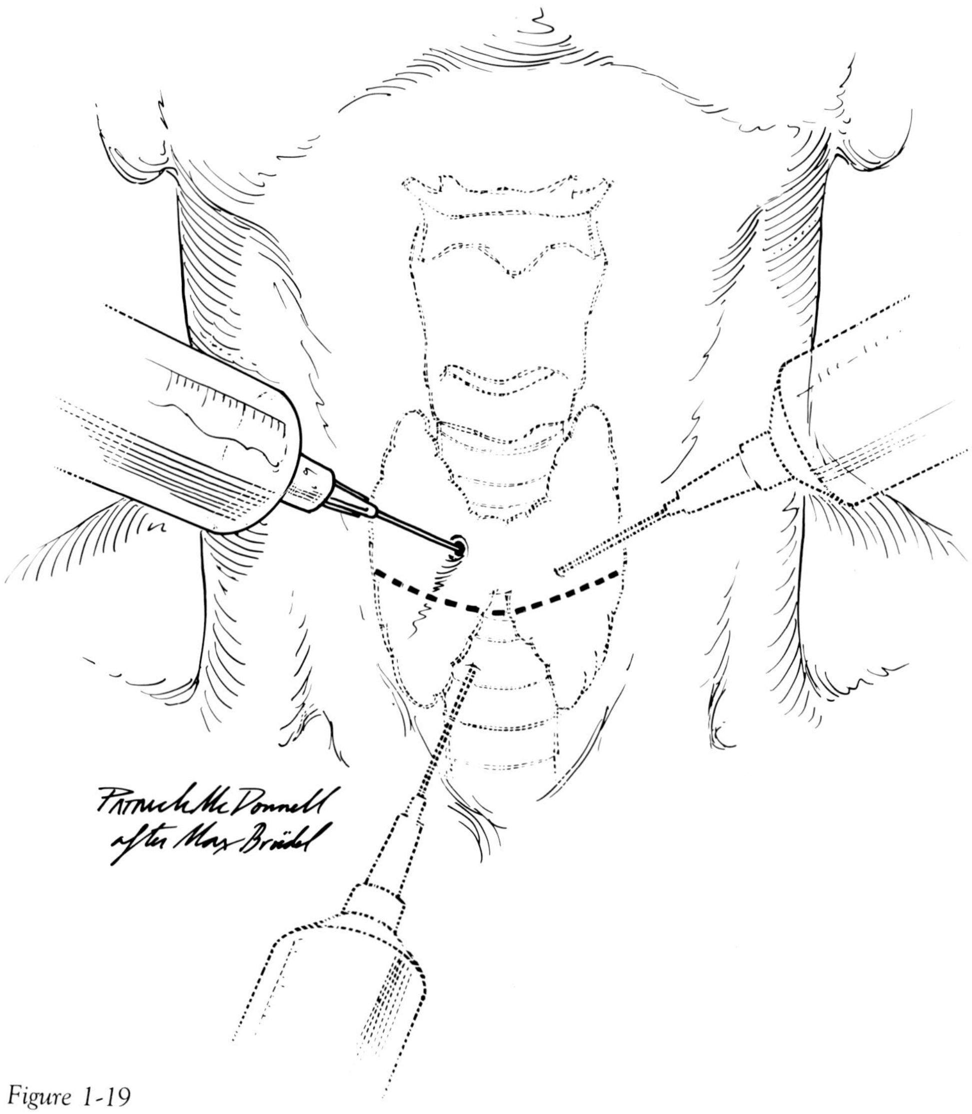

Figure 1-19

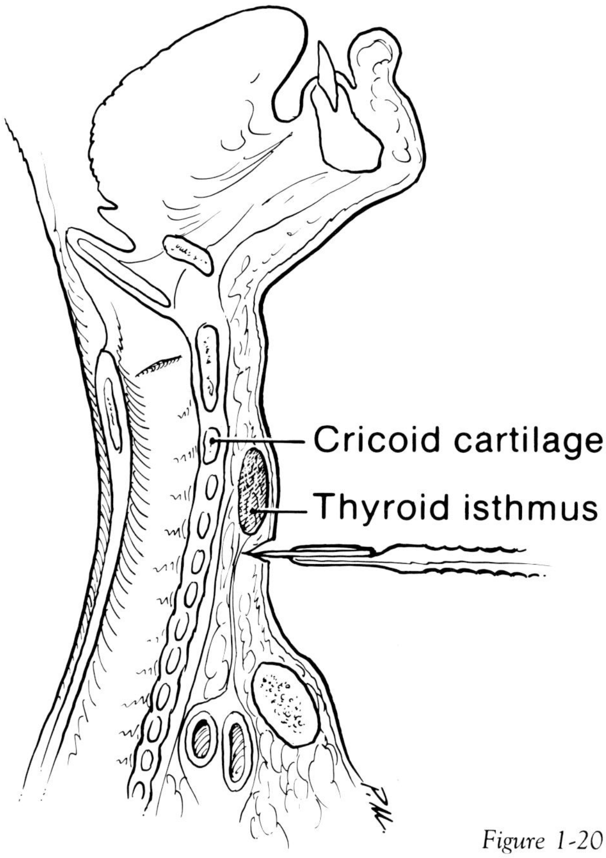

Figure 1-20

A 2–3 cm horizontal incision is made through the skin and subcutaneous tissue until the superficial layer of the cervical fascia is encountered and incised (Figure 1-20).

The investing fascia of the strap muscles is grasped with forceps and incised in the midline with scissors (Figure 1-21).

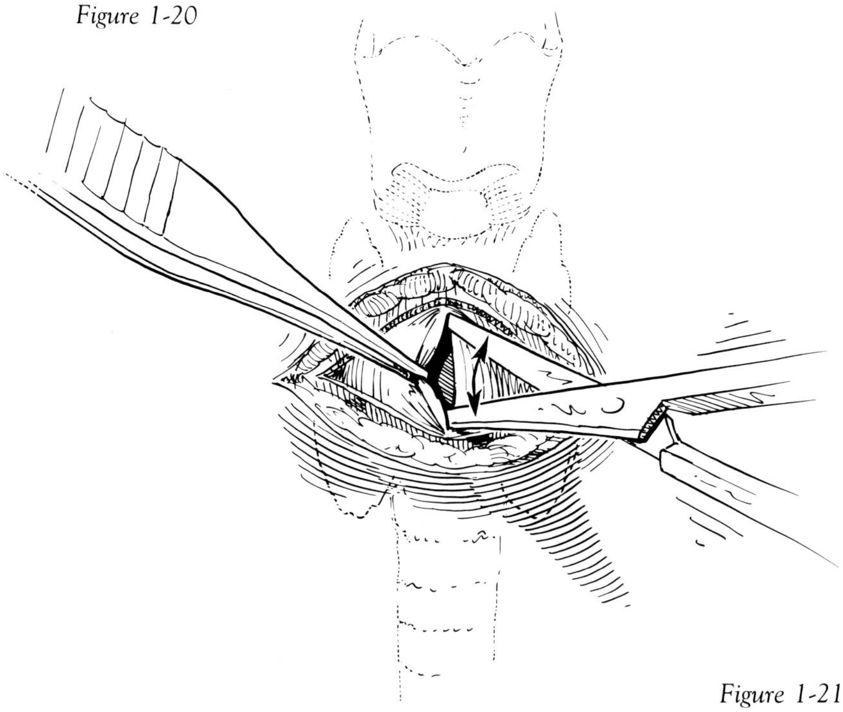

Figure 1-21

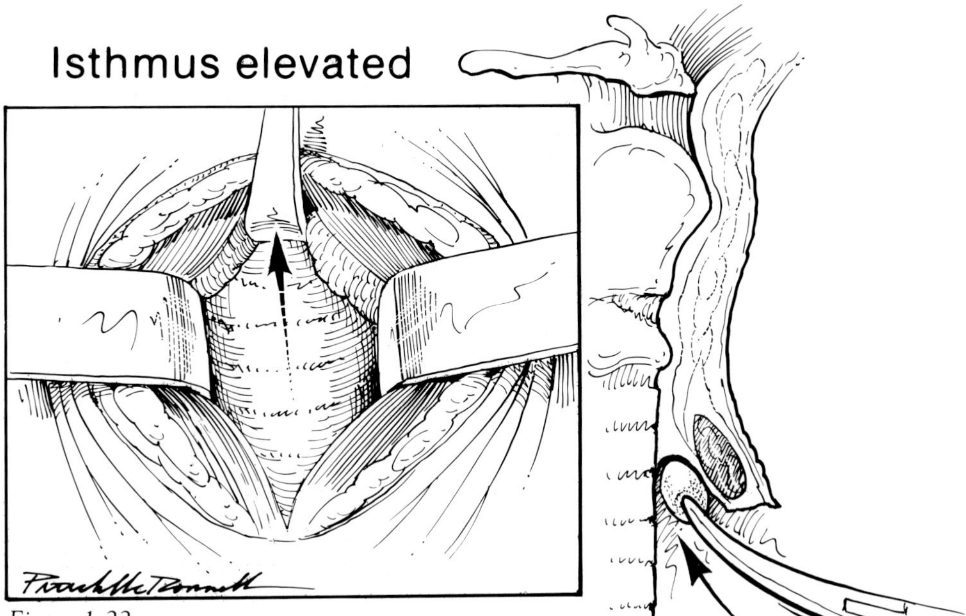

Figure 1-22

The strap muscles are retracted laterally (Figure 1-22). The dissection is carried down to the level of the trachea, inferior to the isthmus of the thyroid gland. The pretracheal fascia is incised, and with a clamp or a Kittner dissector, the thyroid gland is elevated off the anterior surface of the trachea in a plane just deep to the pretracheal fascia.

The cricoid ring is palpated anteriorly, and each tracheal ring is carefully palpated until the interspace between the second and third tracheal ring is encountered (Figure 1-23).

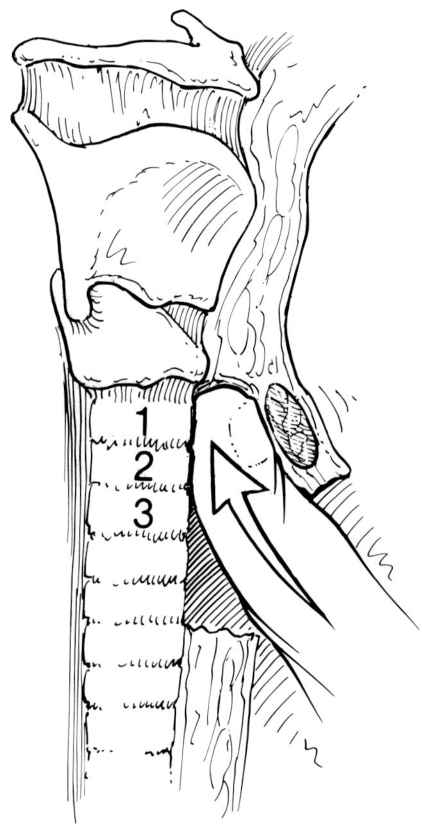

Figure 1-23

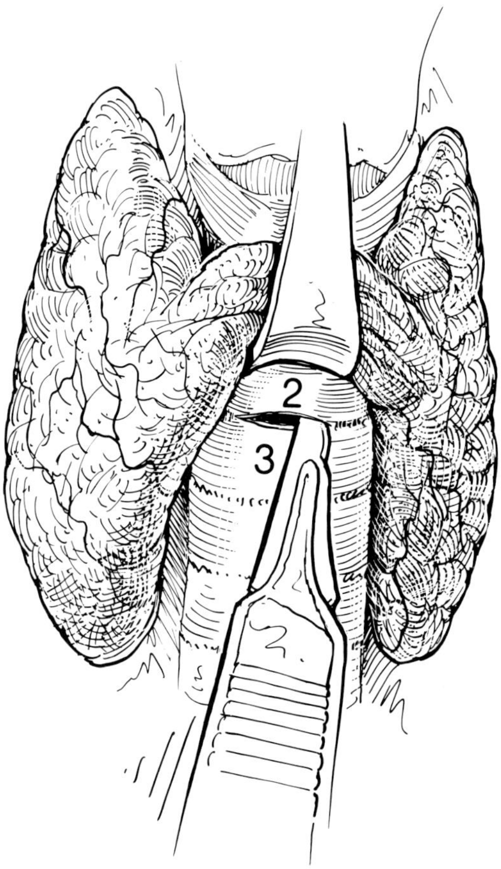

Figure 1-24

A horizontal incision is made through the interspace between the second and third rings using a No. 15 blade (Figure 1-24). In the patient with a laryngeal injury, a more inferior tracheotomy should be considered to avoid the traumatized area.

The inferior tracheal edge is grasped with an Allis clamp (Figure 1-25). Incisions are made inferiorly with either a No. 15 blade or Mayo scissors to create an inferiorly based U-shaped flap of the trachea. (This flap can be replaced when the tracheotomy tube is removed, thereby reducing the chance of stenosis.)

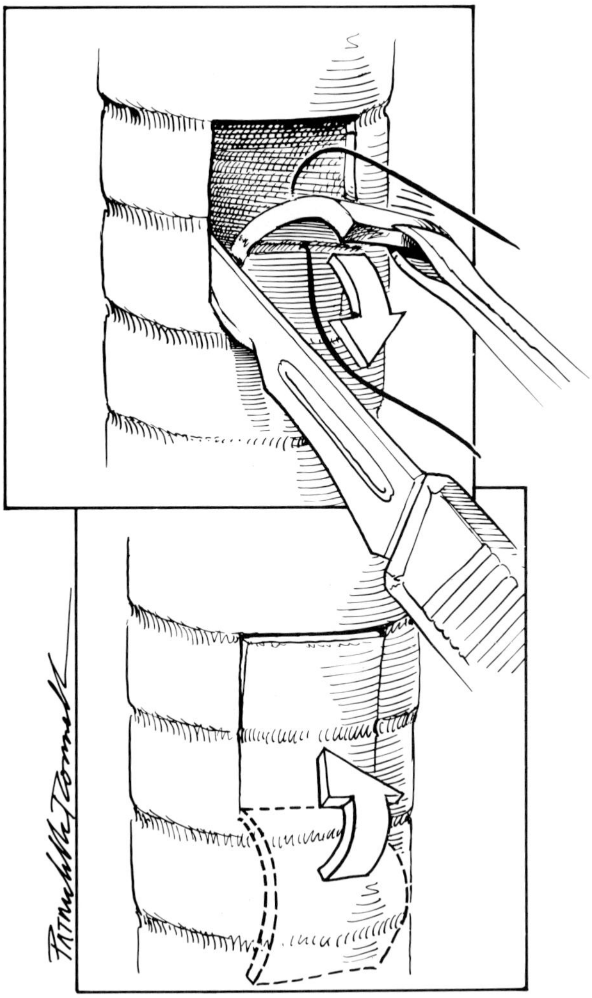

Figure 1-25

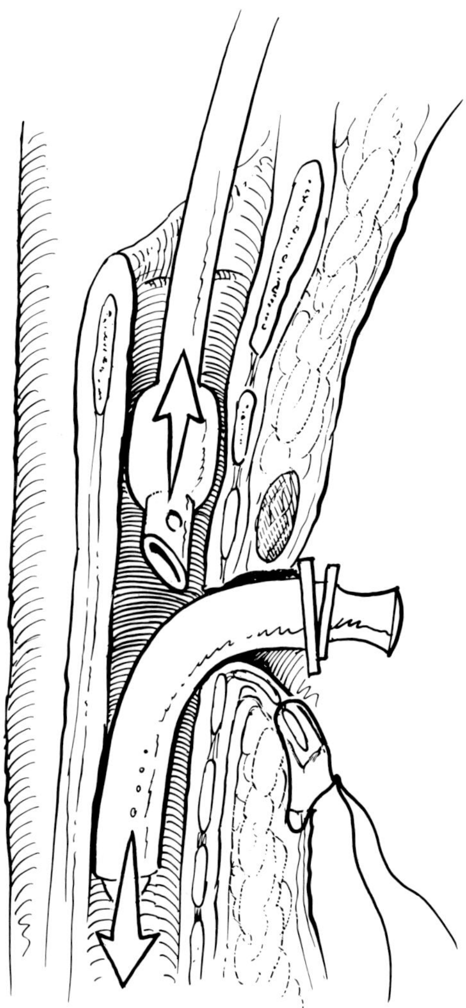

Figure 1-26

A 3-0 silk suture is then passed through the inferior skin edge and the tracheal flap and loosely tied to facilitate retraction of the tracheal flap (Figure 1-26). Under direct visualization the endotracheal tube is carefully withdrawn until the tip of the tube is just above the tracheotomy site and the tracheotomy tube is inserted. A prefabricated dressing is placed around the tracheotomy tube, which is secured by the tape tied around the neck.

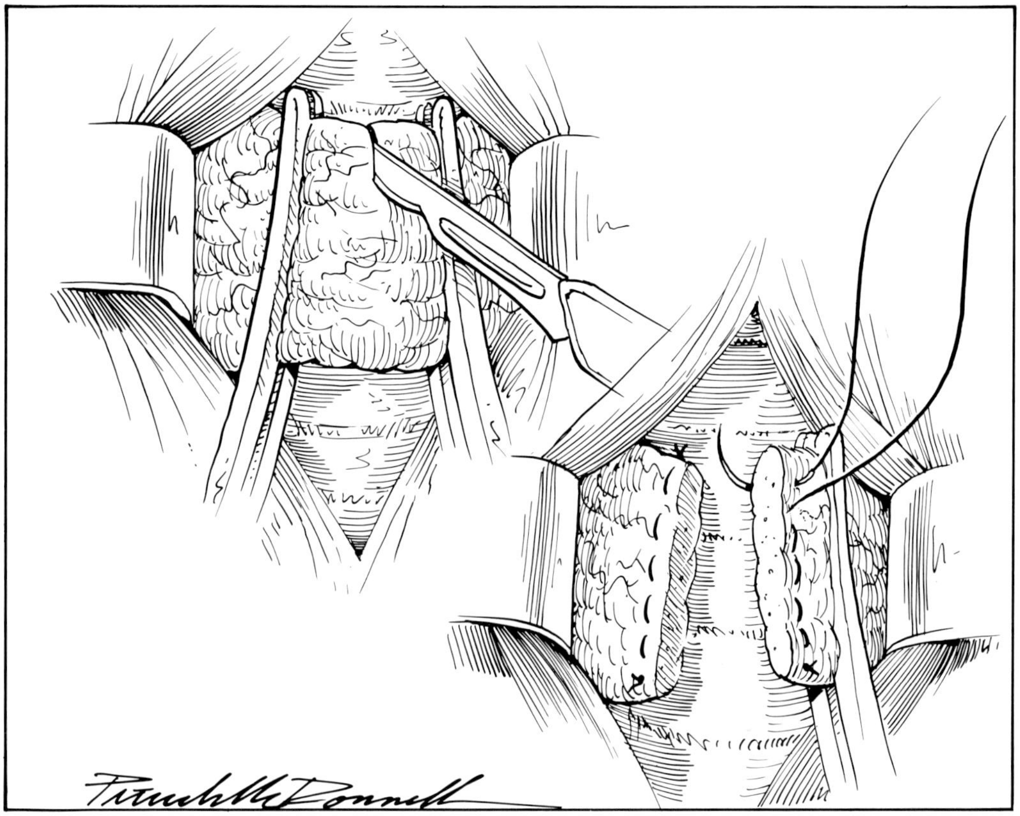

Figure 1-27

ALTERNATIVE TECHNIQUES AND SPECIAL CASES

In cases where the isthmus of the thyroid gland is quite large it may be necessary to divide the thyroid gland. This is accomplished by passing two clamps around the isthmus, which is then divided with a scalpel (Figure 1-27). A chromic suture is sewn in a running fashion over the cut edges of the gland, and the clamps are removed.

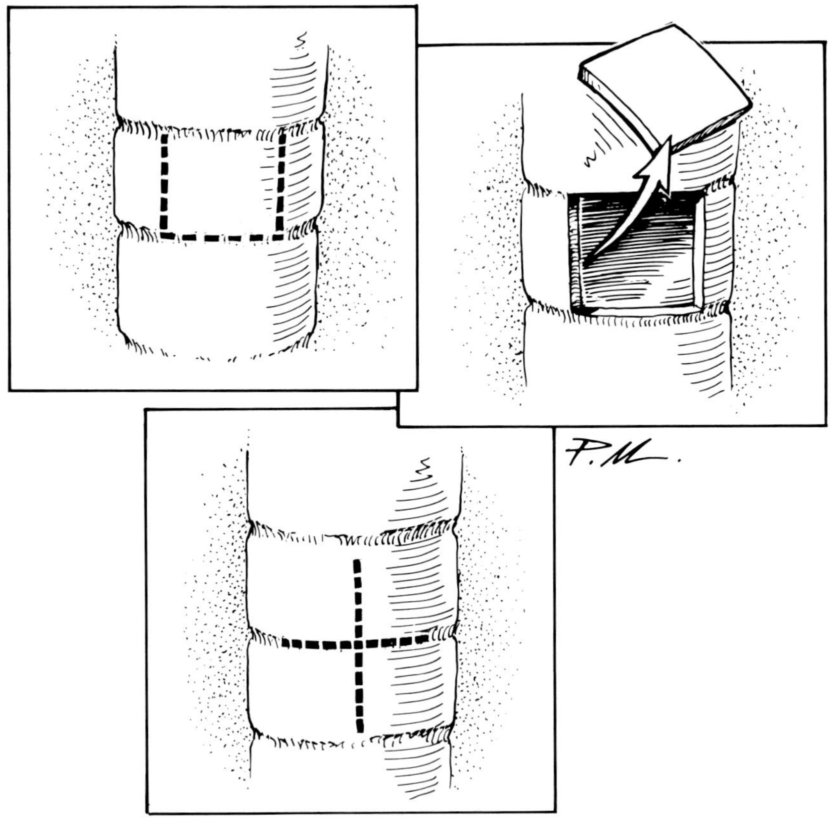

Figure 1-28

Alternative tracheal openings include a superiorly based flap, removal of a cartilaginous "window," and a cruciate incision (Figure 1-28).

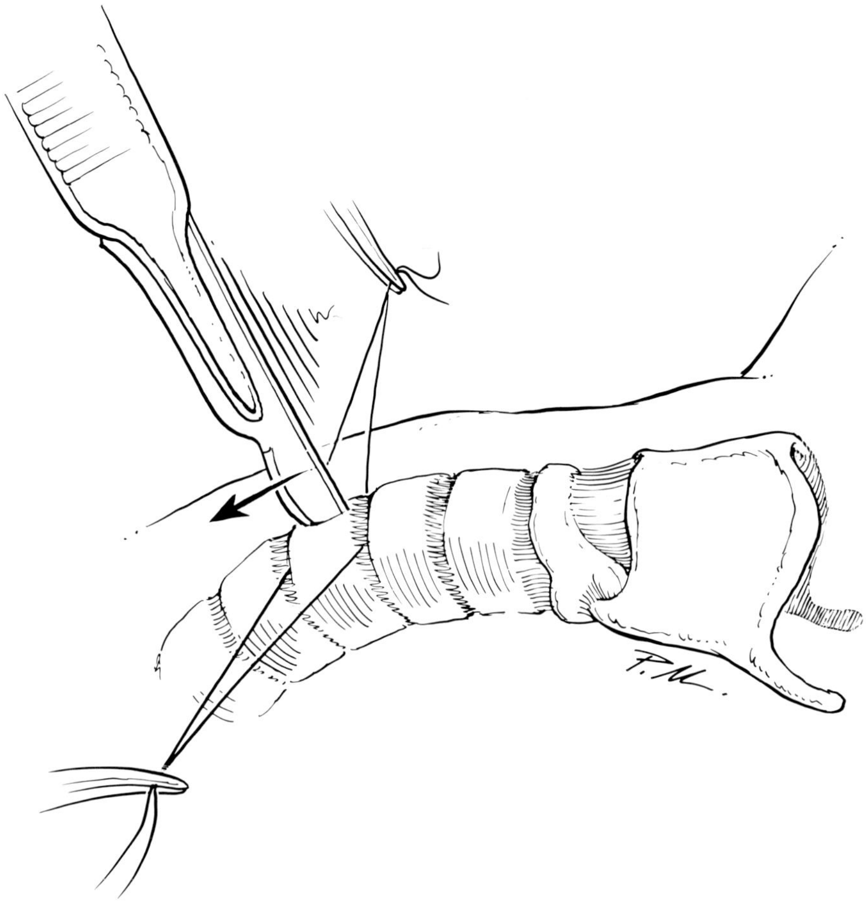

Figure 1-29

Tracheotomy in the pediatric patient is performed in a similar fashion, although many surgeons prefer a vertical midline incision in the trachea rather than a flap (Figure 1-29). A 4-0 silk suture is passed around the third tracheal ring on both sides of the planned incision site. A vertical incision is then made between the sutures.

In infants and very young children, the author prefers to sew the initial tracheotomy tube to the cervical skin in addition to the usual tracheotomy tape passed around the neck (Figure 1-30). The sutures around the tracheal rings are left in place until the first tube is changed at 1 week, so that if the tracheotomy tube becomes dislodged, the sutures can be used as guides for reinsertion of the tracheotomy tube.

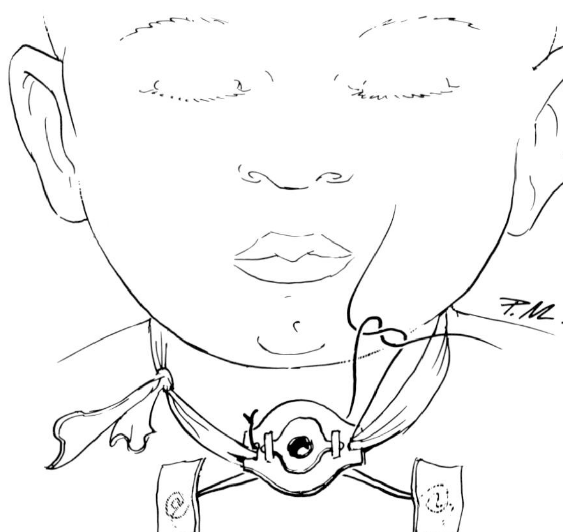

Figure 1-30

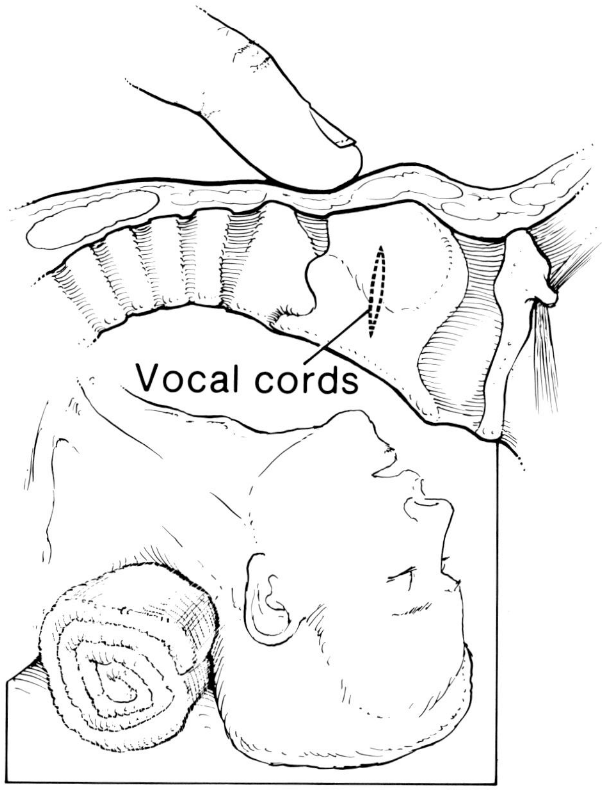

Figure 1-31

CRICOTHYROIDOTOMY

Although there is debate regarding the use of cricothyroidotomy for prolonged airway management, this technique is certainly useful in the emergency situation, particularly if one is not familiar with the technique of tracheotomy.

A roll is placed under the patient's shoulders to extend the neck, and the space between the cricoid and the thyroid cartilages is palpated (Figure 1-31).

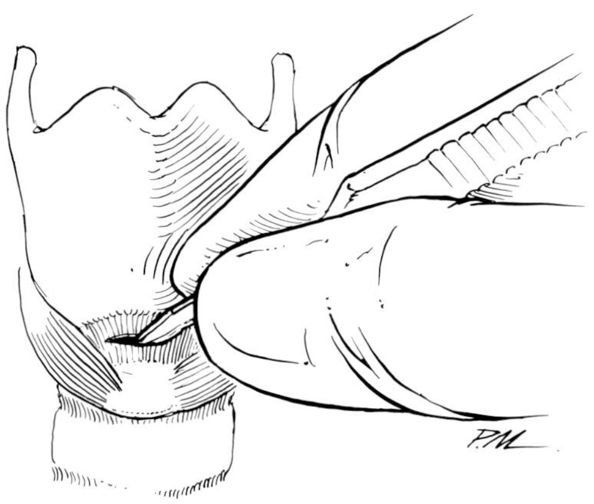

Figure 1-32

A horizontal incision through the skin and the cricothyroid membrane is created using a No. 15 blade (Figure 1-32).

A small hemostat is placed in the wound, and the cricoid and thyroid cartilages are gently separated anteriorly (Figure 1-33).

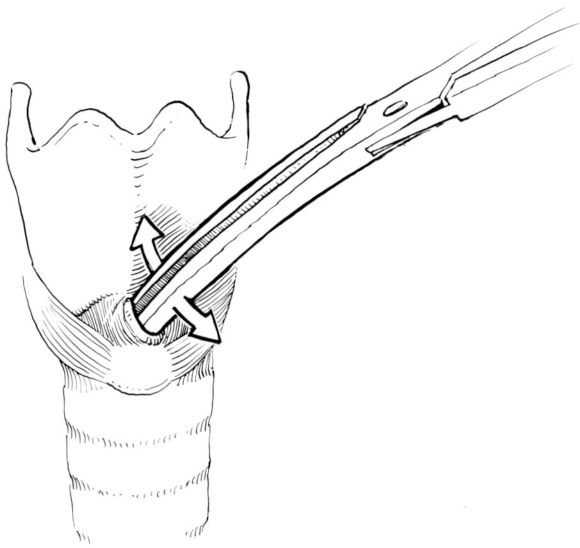

Figure 1-33

Heavy Mayo scissors are then used to spread the cricothyroid membrane horizontally until a tracheotomy tube can be inserted (Figure 1-34).

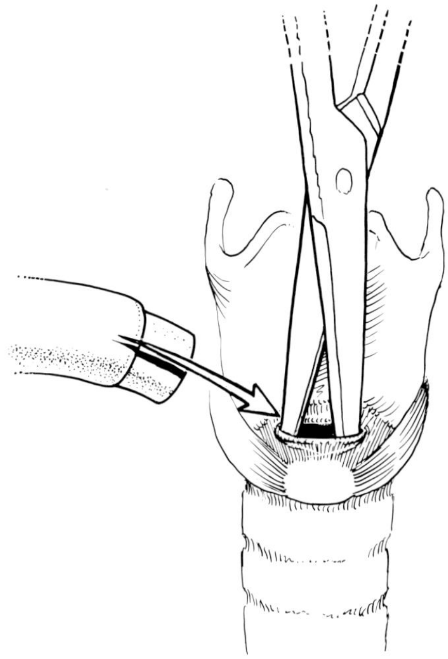

Figure 1-34

REFERENCES

1. Brantigan, C. O. and Grow, J. B.: Cricothyroidotomy: Elective Use in Respiratory Problems Requiring Tracheotomy. *J. Thorac. Cardiovasc. Surg.*, 71:72–81, 1976.
2. Lulenski, G. C.: Long-term Tracheal Dimensions After Flap Tracheostomy. *Arch. Otolaryngol.*, 107:114–116, 1981.
3. Lulenski, G. C. and Batsakis, J. G.: Management of the Flap Tracheostomy. *Arch. Otolaryngol.*, 105:260–263, 1979.

2

Fractures of the Mandible

David W. Shelton

INITIAL STABILIZATION

Any technique that immobilizes the fractured mandible against the intact maxilla will effectively stabilize the fracture and make the patient more comfortable.

The simplest method of providing some immediate support for the fractured mandible is a head bandage (Figure 2-1). A disadvantage is that it may displace mobile fractures of the mandible posteriorly, resulting in increased bleeding and possible airway compromise. These dressings are easily displaced and provide little real support for the fracture. They may be used temporarily for patient comfort but should not be placed tightly over grossly mobile fractures.

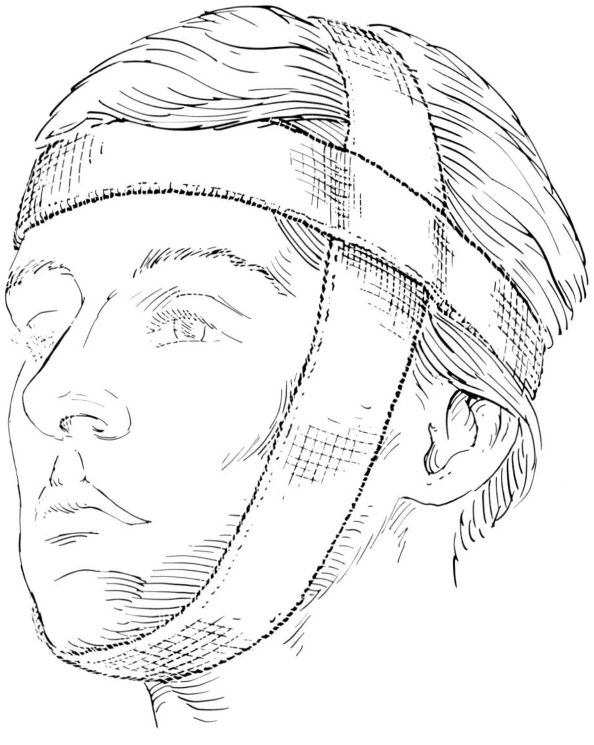

Figure 2-1

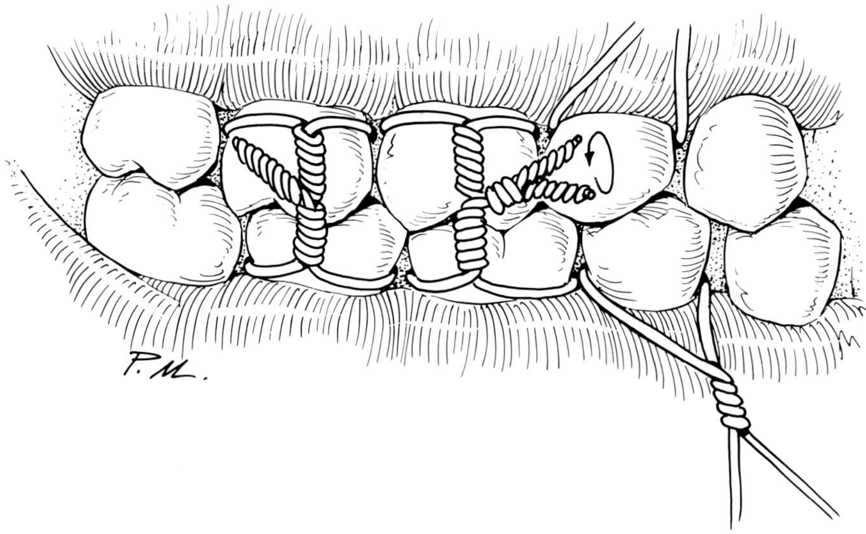

Figure 2-2

GILMER METHOD

After local anesthesia is obtained, the opposing maxillary and mandibular teeth are individually ligated circumferentially and the free ends of the wire are twisted together (Figure 2-2). The teeth are brought into occlusion and secured by opposing free cables twisted together.

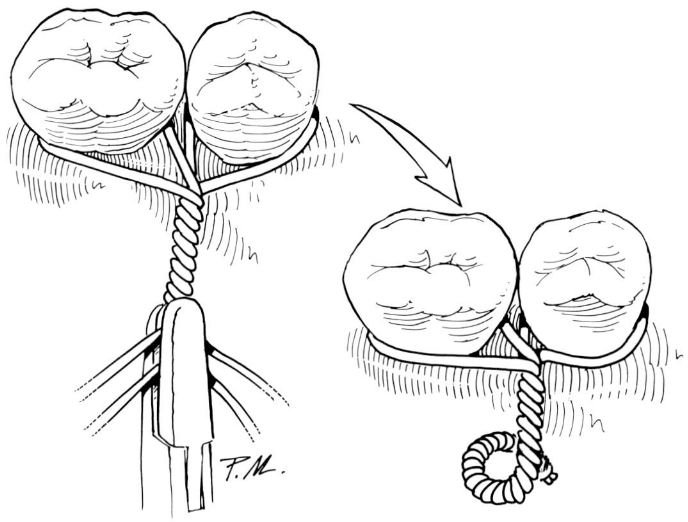

Figure 2-3

KAZANJIAN BUTTON

After local anesthesia is obtained, adjacent teeth are individually ligated circumferentially with 24-gauge stainless steel wire, and the free ends of both ligatures are twisted together and formed into a rosette (Figure 2-3).

The teeth are brought into occlusion and secured by applying either intermaxillary wires or elastics utilizing opposing rosettes as anchorage (Figure 2-4).

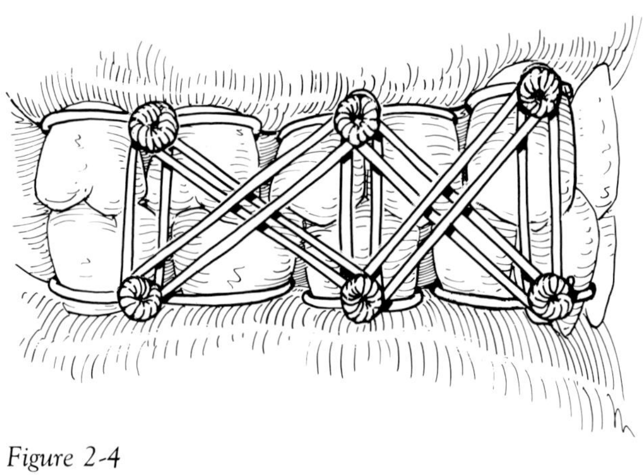

Figure 2-4

EYELET LOOP

An 8-cm length of 24-gauge stainless steel wire is cut and doubled upon itself. A small loop is formed at the bend in the wire and twisted two turns. The free ends of the wire are passed between adjacent teeth and advanced to the twists of the loop (Figure 2-5). The free ends are then passed in opposite directions circumferentially around the adjacent teeth. The free end of the posterior wire is then directed through the loop and twisted with the anterior wire until the arrangement is secure. A similar configuration is placed in the opposing dental arch. The loops may then be bent toward the occlusal plane to receive an intermaxillary wire, or away from the occlusal plane to serve as anchorage for intermaxillary elastics. In selected mandibular fractures, many well-placed eyelet loops, either alone or in conjunction with internal fixation, may serve as definitive treatment.

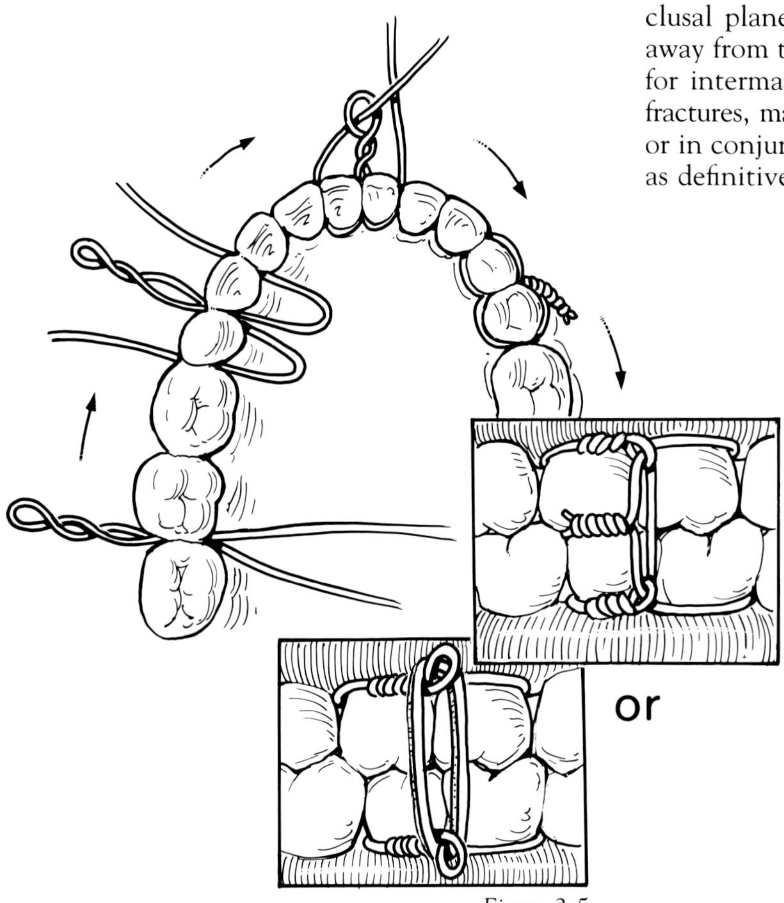

Figure 2-5

DEFINITIVE INTERMAXILLARY FIXATION

STOUT METHOD

A 24-cm length of 24-gauge stainless steel wire is passed around the last molar tooth and placed against the buccal and lingual aspects of the teeth (Figure 2-6).

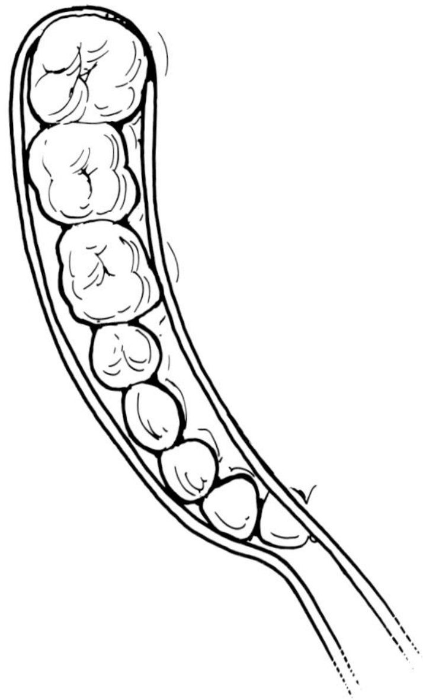

Figure 2-6

The lingual wire is passed through the dental embrasure, around the buccal wire, and back through the same embrasure (Figure 2-7).

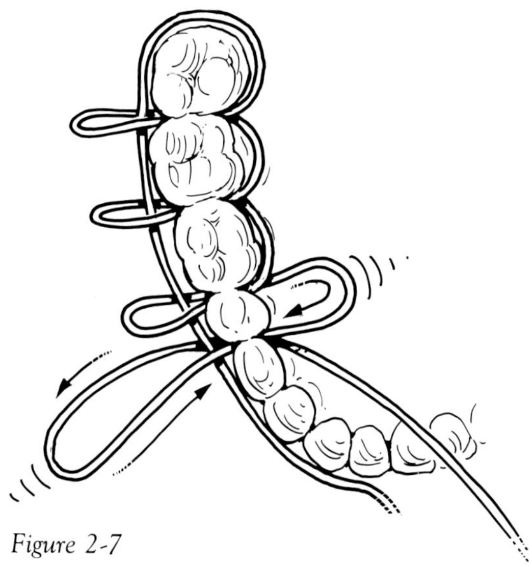

Figure 2-7

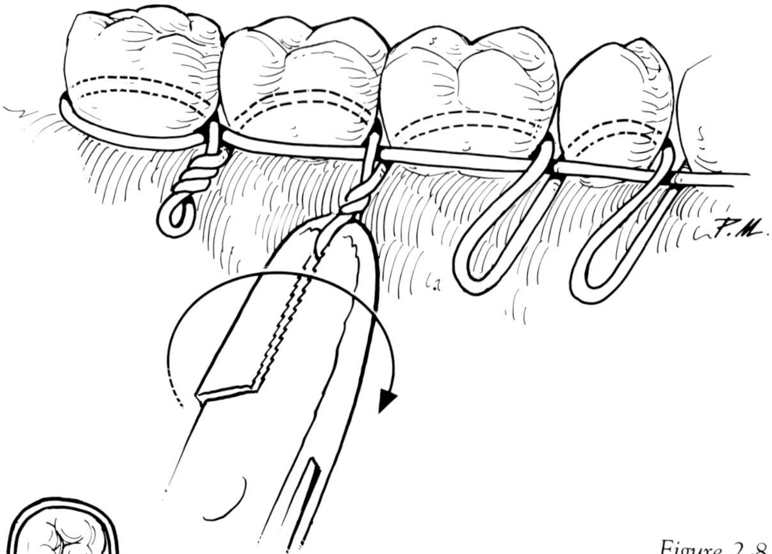

Figure 2-8

A loop is then formed and twisted until the arrangement is secure (Figure 2-8). There should be no more than two or three twists behind the loop. The wiring procedures are repeated in sequence about each succeeding tooth in the dental arch and terminated at the cuspid tooth by twisting the wire emerging through the embrasure with the free end of the buccal wire.

The procedure is carried out in the opposing dentition bilaterally (Figure 2-9).

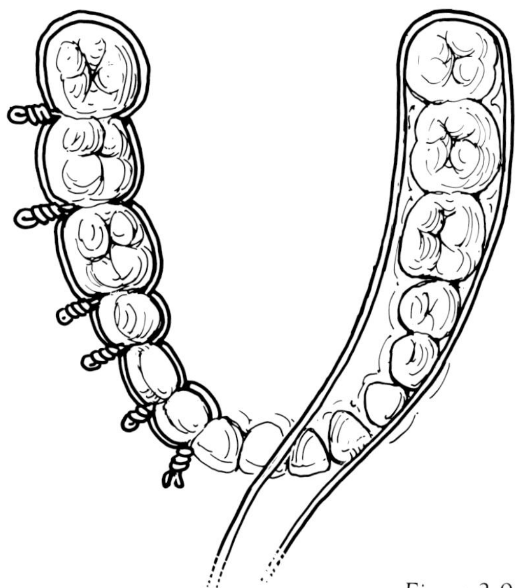

Figure 2-9

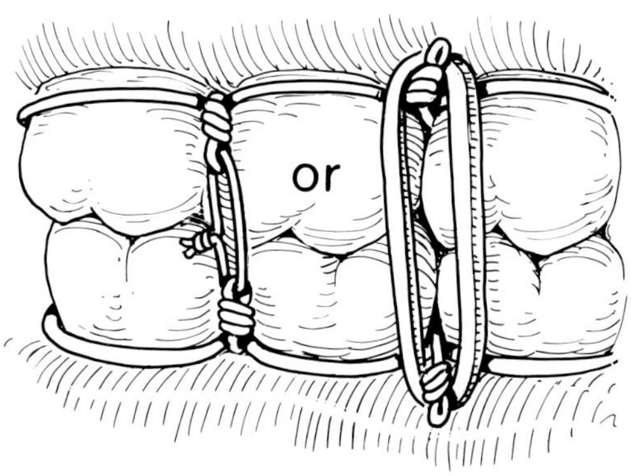

Figure 2-10

The loops may then be turned toward the occlusal plane to receive an intermaxillary wire or away from the occlusal plane to serve as anchorage for intermaxillary elastics (Figure 2-10).

ARCH BARS

A stock arch bar is measured and cut to the appropriate length by being laid around the buccolabial circumference of the dental arch at the level of the necks of the teeth (Figure 2-11). The posterior extent of the arch bar is inclined inward to engage the distal curvature of the last molar tooth.

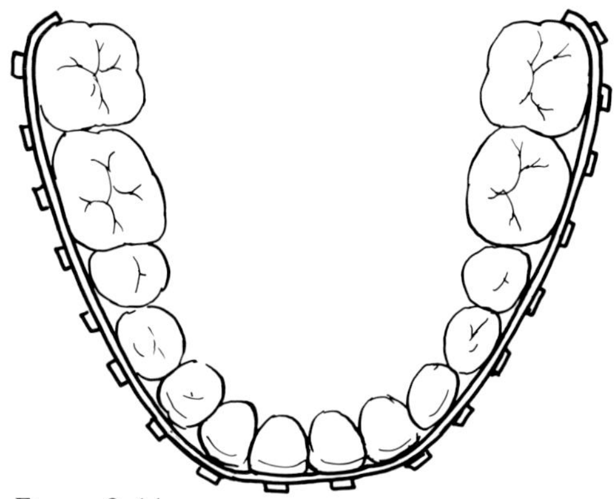

Figure 2-11

A 24-gauge stainless steel wire is passed through the embrasures of the second bicuspid, above the arch bar on one side and below on the other (Figure 2-12). A gauze-packing instrument is used to push the lingual wire toward the root of the tooth as the wire is tightened. Initial fixation of the arch bar to both bicuspids anchors the arch bar in place and facilitates the placement of subsequent ligature wires.

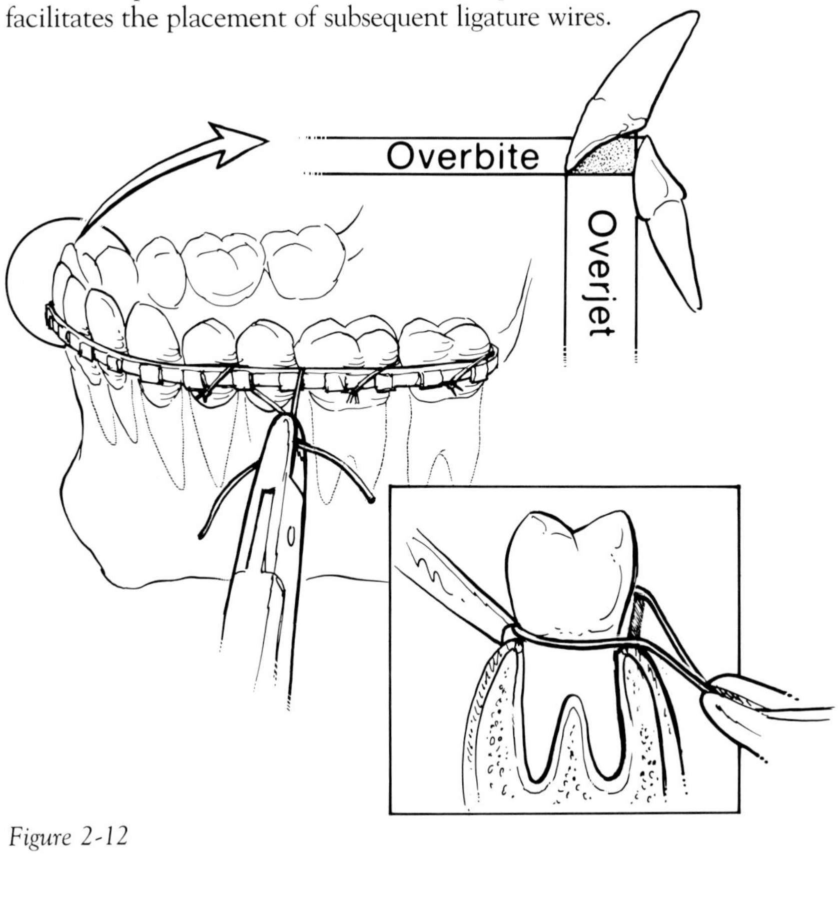

Figure 2-12

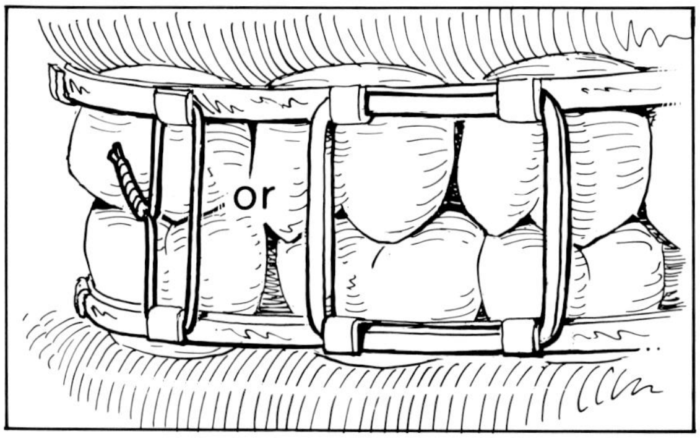

Figure 2-13

The arch bar is similarly ligated to as many teeth as necessary to achieve stability. If at least one molar, two premolars, and the cuspid are ligated bilaterally, it is generally unnecessary to ligate the lateral and central incisors. The shape of the crowns of these teeth does not lend itself to good retention of the ligature wire. These teeth also have a single, conical, tapering root and are easily extruded during intermaxillary fixation, especially if they are not in contact with opposing teeth. Frequently the overjet or overbite relationship of the anterior teeth renders placement of effective intermaxillary fixation impractical.

Intermaxillary immobilization of the mandible is then achieved by placing elastics (active traction) or wires (passive fixation) between the lugs of opposing arch bars (Figure 2-13).

DENTAL SPLINTS

The use of dental splints in selected cases is a valuable asset in the management of fractures of the mandible.

Dental casts are made of the patient with a mandibular fracture (Figure 2-14).

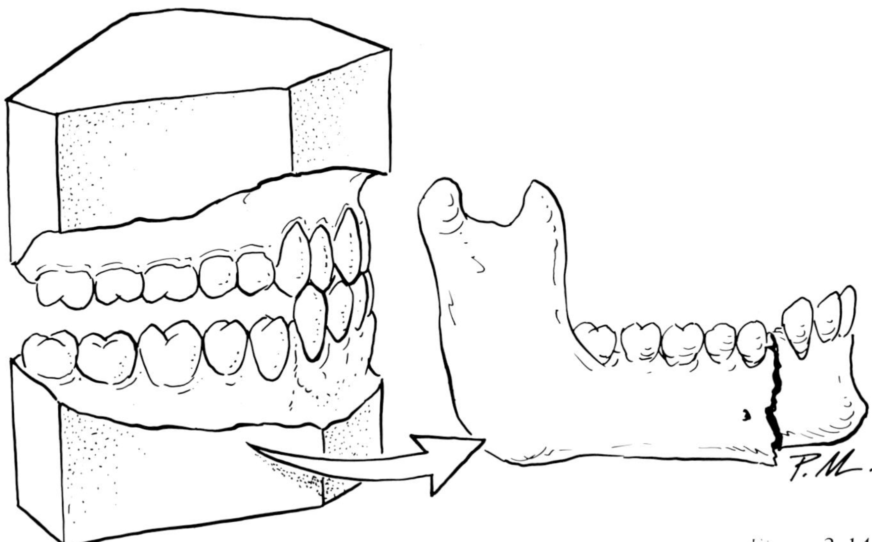

Figure 2-14

The mandibular cast is sectioned along the plane of the fracture as determined from radiographic and clinical examination of the patient (Figure 2-15).

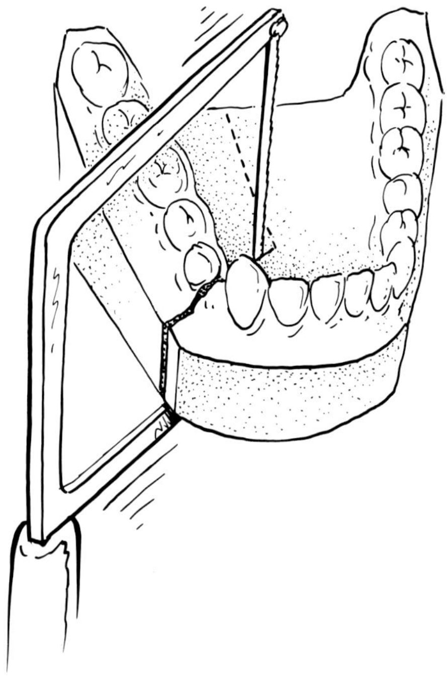

Figure 2-15

The mandibular cast is reassembled in occlusion with the intact maxillary cast, and a new base is applied to fix the reconstructed mandibular cast in its proper position (Figure 2-16).

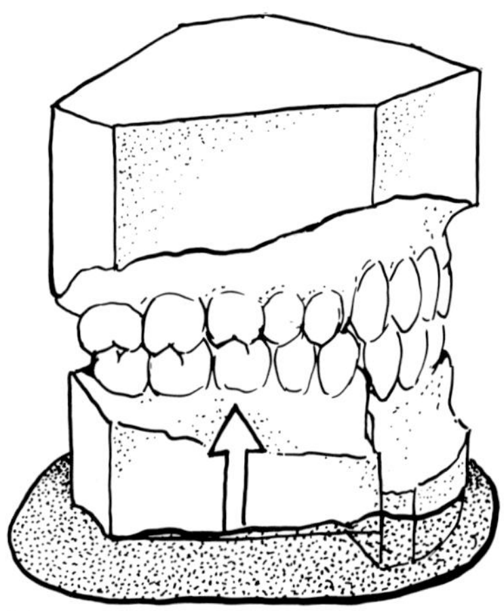

Figure 2-16

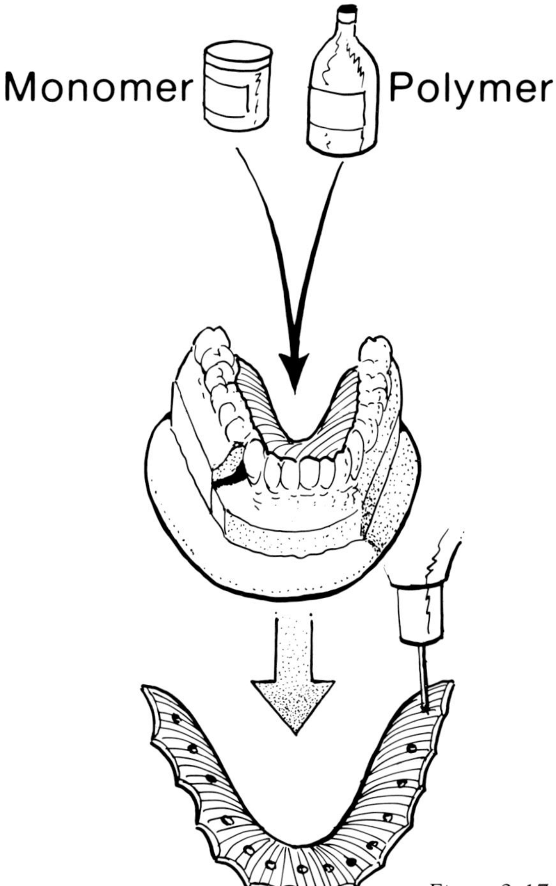

Figure 2-17

Self-curing polymethylmethacrylate acrylic resin (dental acrylic resin) is applied to the lingual aspect of the teeth and alveolar process of the reconstructed mandibular cast (Figure 2-17). After the dental resin is set, the splint is removed from the cast and appropriately trimmed. Holes are placed through the splint to permit the passage of ligature wires.

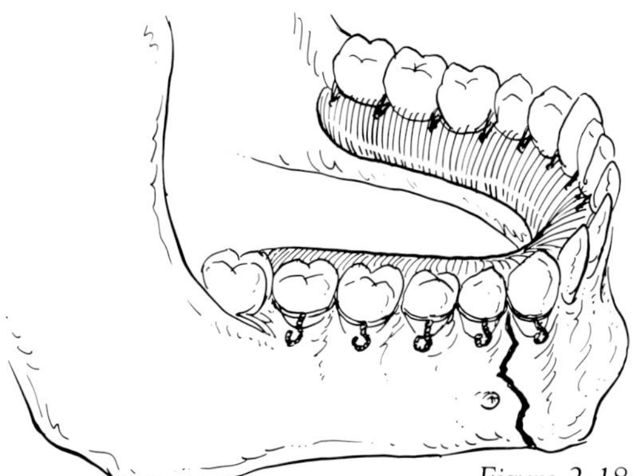
Figure 2-18

The completed splint is placed in the mouth and ligated to the teeth with 24-gauge stainless steel wire (Figure 2-18). The patient is then placed in intermaxillary fixation. All of the steps in the splint process may be performed with the patient under local anesthesia.

ALTERNATIVE TECHNIQUES

Fractures of the alveolar process of the mandible are also well managed with arch bar and splint stabilization.

Smaller dental alveolar fractures, i.e., two to three tooth segments, may be stabilized to an arch bar that has been ligated to adjacent noninvolved teeth (Figure 2-19).

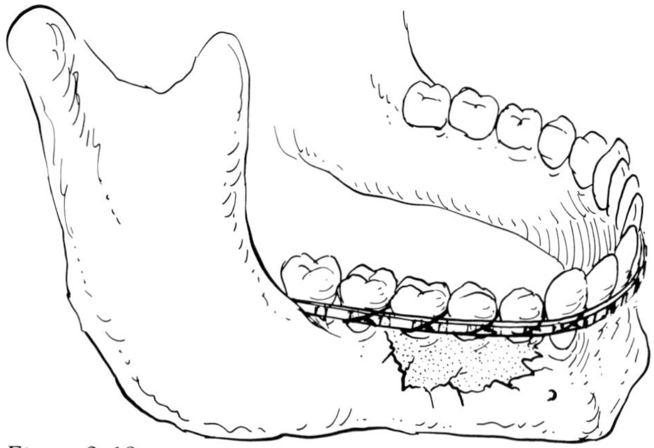

Figure 2-19

Larger dental alveolar fractures generally are best repositioned and stabilized with a splint (Figure 2-20).

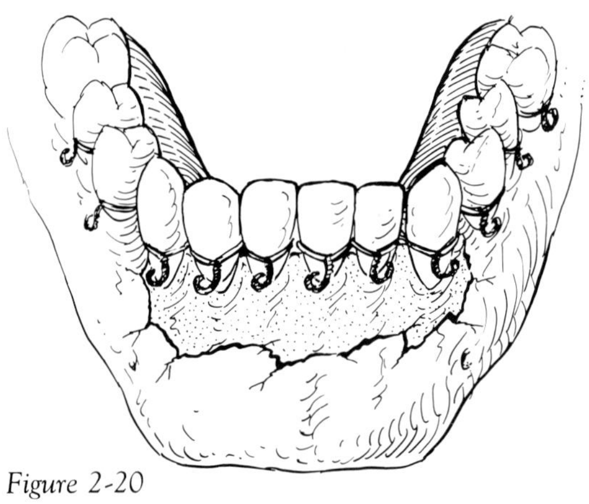

Figure 2-20

INTRAORAL OPEN REDUCTION AND INTERNAL FIXATION

Fractures of the angle of the mandible frequently occur through the third molar tooth socket. Such a situation offers an excellent opportunity to treat a mobile mandibular angle fracture by eliminating a nonfunctional tooth that may be a source of contamination, and simultaneously applying internal fixation to the fractured mandible through an intraoral approach.

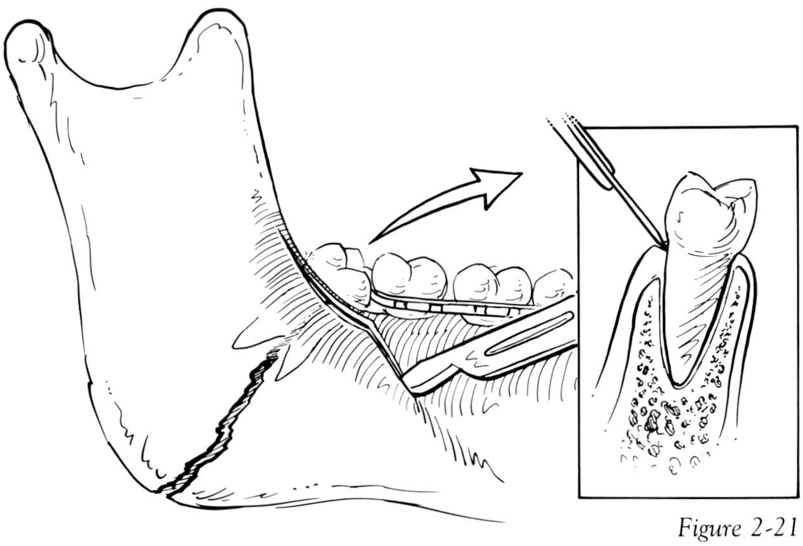

Figure 2-21

The regional soft tissues are infiltrated with 2% lidocaine with epinephrine 1:100,000 to enhance hemostasis. An incision is made over the external oblique ridge of the mandible to the posterior aspect of the third molar tooth to be removed, and continued in the buccogingival crevice of the second molar (Figure 2-21). A vertical oblique relaxing incision is made at the anterior aspect of the second molar. The mucoperiosteum is reflected from the lateral aspect of the mandible, and the mandibular angle fracture is visualized along the lateral cortex and at the alveolar crest.

The mandibular third molar tooth is removed, and the teeth are brought into occlusion (Figure 2-22). Temporary wires are passed around the arch bars to maintain the occlusion. Under direct vision the posterior fragment is aligned anatomically with the anterior fragment, and the location of the bur holes is marked on both the posterior and anterior fragments.

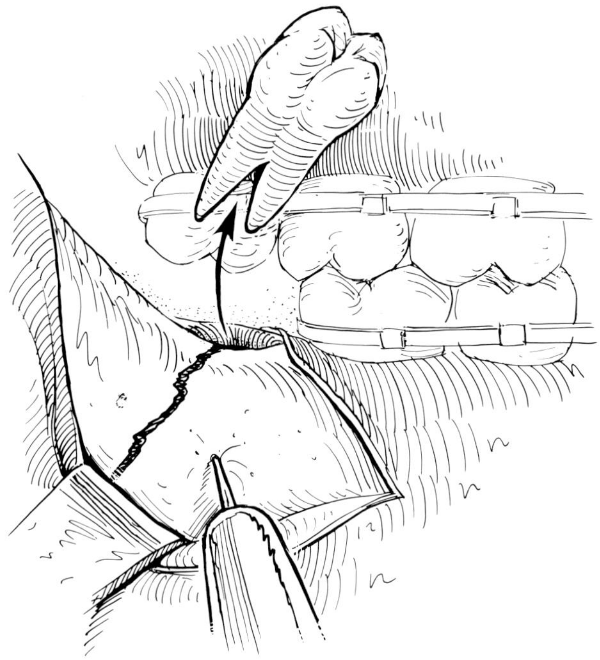

Figure 2-22

The mouth is opened after the temporary wires are cut, and bur holes are placed through the lateral cortical bone of both posterior and anterior fragments into the tooth socket at the locations previously marked (Figure 2-23).

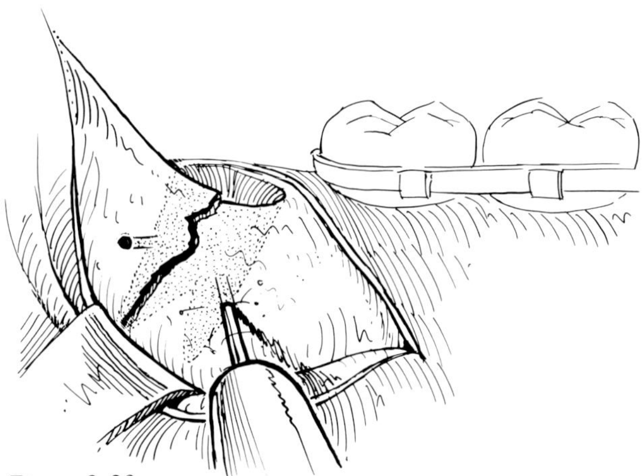

Figure 2-23

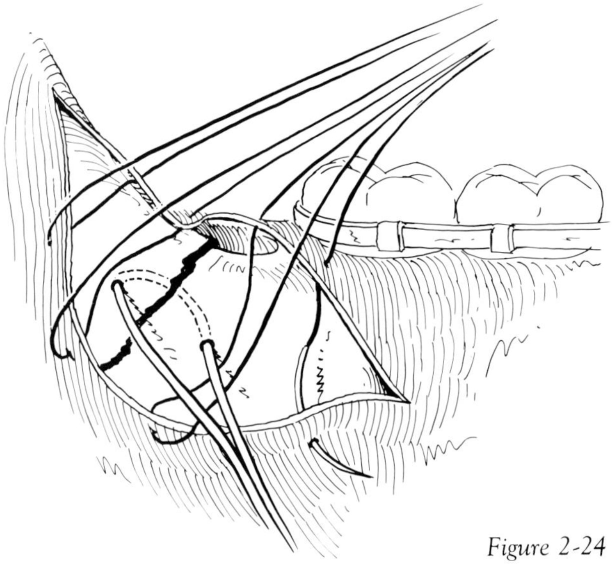

A 24-gauge stainless steel wire is passed through the hole, brought loosely out of the mouth, and tagged with a clamp (Figure 2-24). Then 4-0 chromic sutures are placed across the incision and also brought loosely out of the mouth and tagged with a clamp.

Figure 2-24

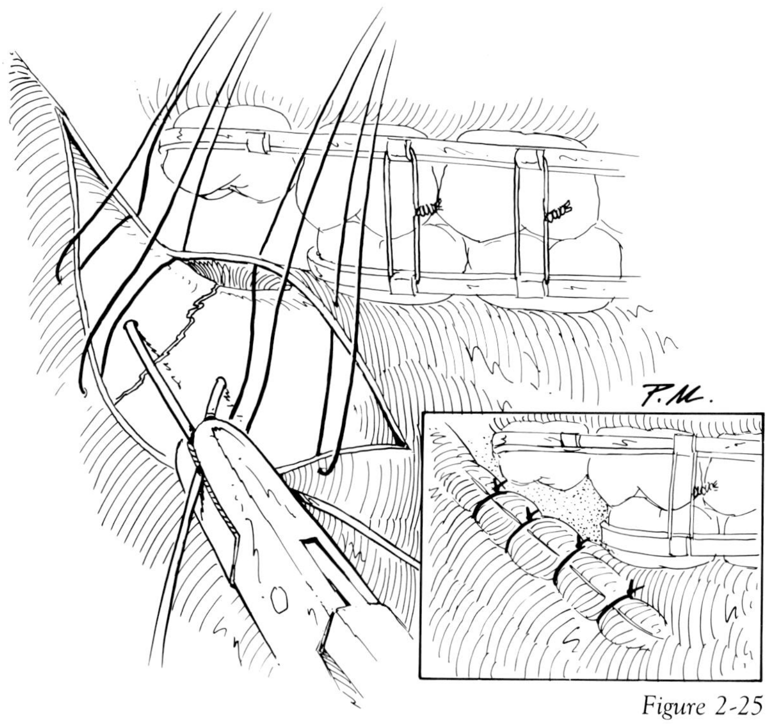

Figure 2-25

The teeth are brought into occlusion and intermaxillary fixation is achieved (Figure 2-25). The posterior fragment is again aligned anatomically with the anterior fragment under direct vision, and the internal fixation wire is tightened. The sutures are tied and the incision is closed.

EXTERNAL OPEN REDUCTION AND INTERNAL FIXATION

The patient is placed on the operating table in a supine position. A towel roll is placed under the shoulders to moderately extend the head, thereby lifting the chin and mandible away from the chest. Prior to preparation of the face the regional tissues in the operative area are infiltrated with epinephrine 1:100,000. Lidocaine-containing solutions are avoided due to the possibility of blocking the mandibular ramus of the facial nerve. The angle region of the mandible is draped in a fashion that exposes the areas supplied by the mandibular ramus of the facial nerve. If there is no opposing occlusion in the posterior fragment, the teeth may be fixed in occlusion at the beginning of the procedure and only the posterior fragment manipulated at the time of surgery.

A curvilinear horizontal incision is made 2–3 cm below the inferior border of the mandible and carried sharply to the level of the platysma (Figure 2-26). Location of the incision is determined from preoperative clinical and radiographic examinations.

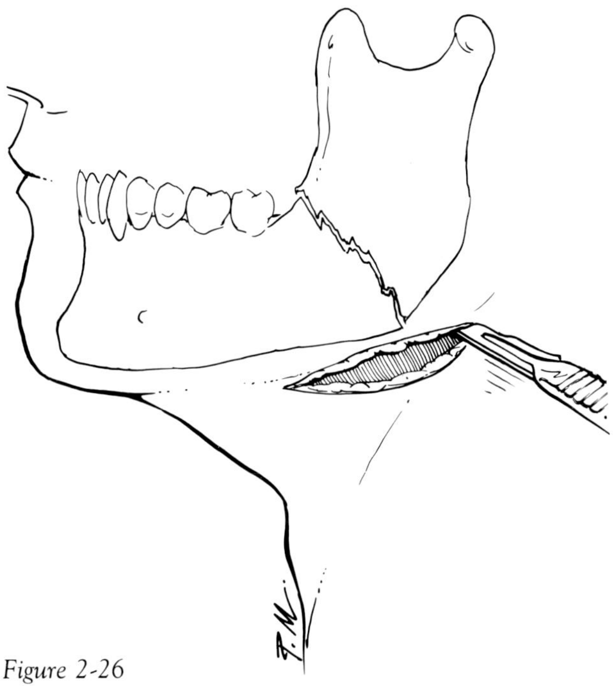

Figure 2-26

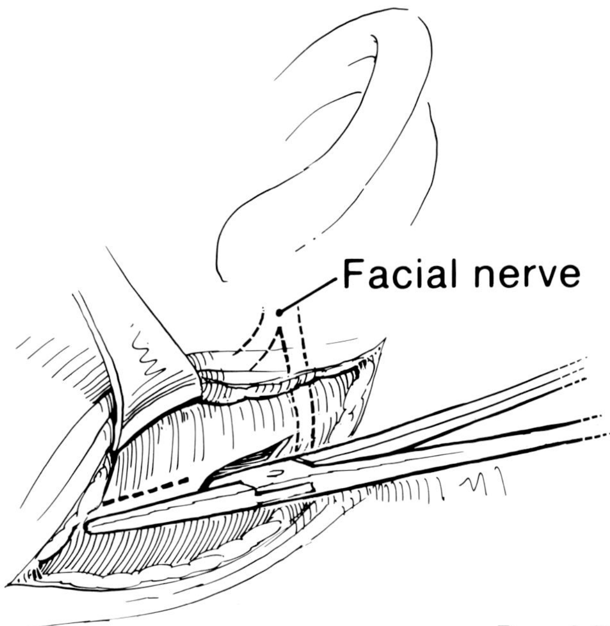

Figure 2-27

The tissue plane immediately below the platysma muscle is entered at the anterior or posterior aspect of the incision and undermined (Figure 2-27). One blade of a straight mosquito hemostat is inserted below the platysma muscle and one above it. The muscle is gently squeezed to check that the marginal mandibular nerve is not in the area, and then it is sharply divided. A nerve stimulator can also be used to identify the nerve.

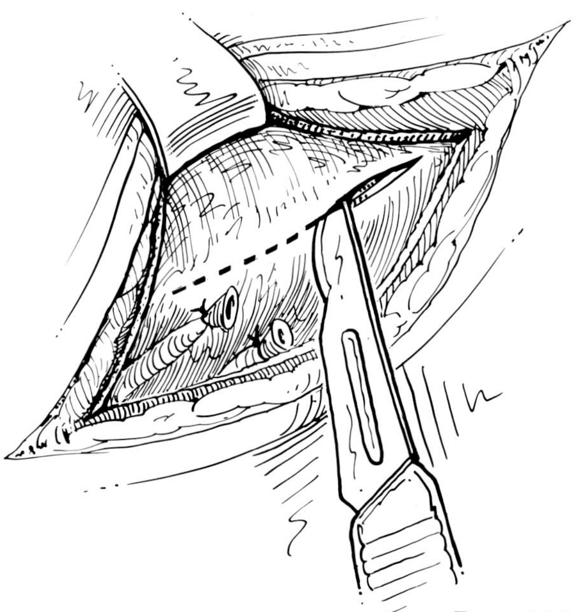

Figure 2-28

The facial artery and vein are isolated, divided, and ligated (Figure 2-28). If the marginal mandibular nerve is uncovered in the dissection, it is isolated and protected. The inferior border of the mandible is approached by alternate sharp and blunt dissection. The periosteum is incised along the inferior border of the mandible, exposing the fracture.

The periosteum and masseter muscles are elevated from the lateral surface of the mandible, exposing the fracture (Figure 2-29). It is also necessary to elevate the periosteum over the medial surface of the mandible, although less extensively.

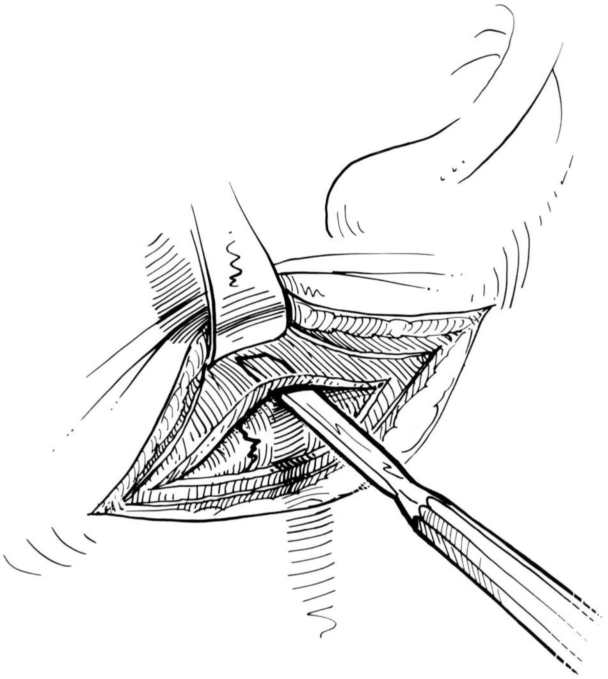

Figure 2-29

The posterior fragment is grasped with bone-holding forceps and distracted inferiorly and laterally (Figure 2-30). Tissue debris interposed in the fracture line is curetted to permit approximation of the fragments.

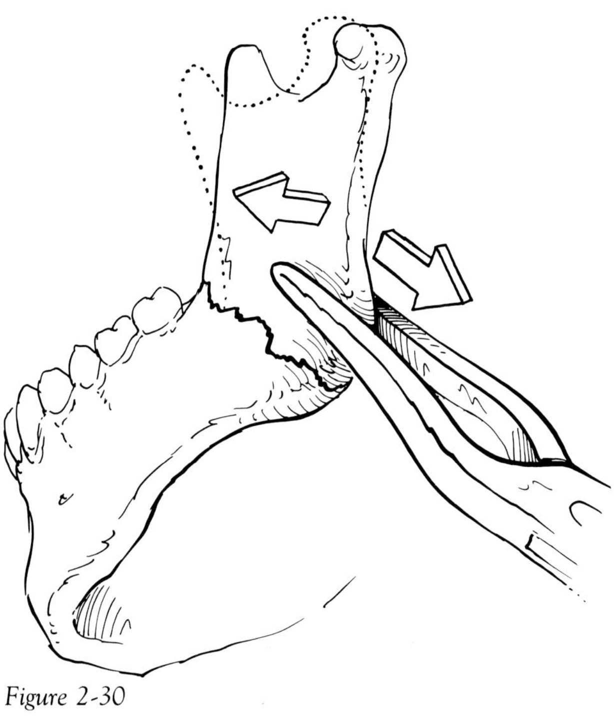

Figure 2-30

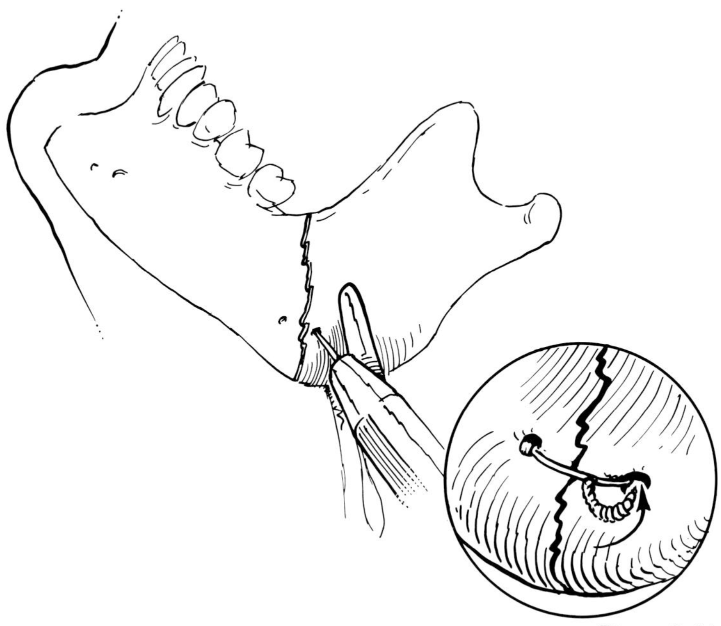

Figure 2-31

With the fracture held in reduction, bur holes are placed through the bone 0.5–1 cm on either side of the fracture (Figure 2-31). The bur holes are placed so that an internal fixation wire will cross the plane of fracture at a right angle. Additional bur holes and wires may be placed as deemed necessary. The free ends of the wire are twisted, cut, and bent into one of the bur holes.

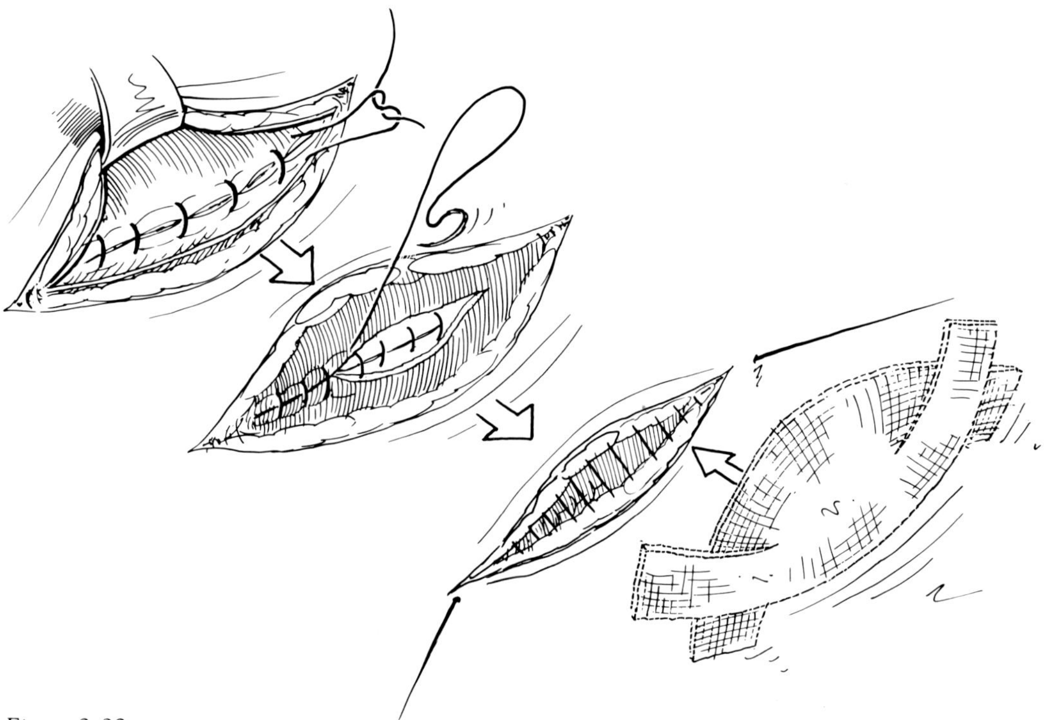

Figure 2-32

The pterygomasseteric muscular sling and periosteum are closed with absorbable sutures (Figure 2-32). The skin is closed in a subcuticular fashion. A light pressure dressing is then applied utilizing elastic tape.

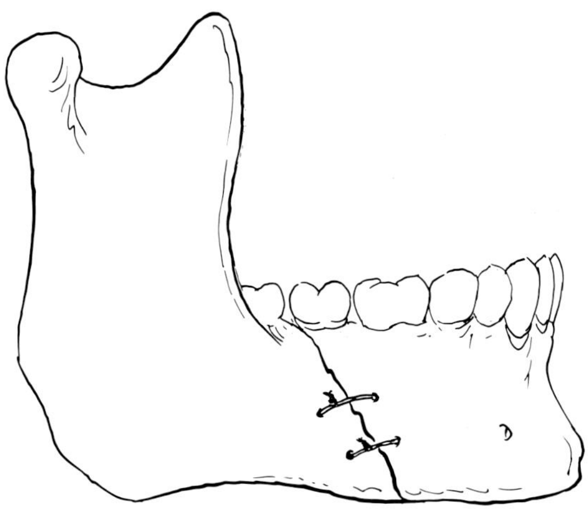

Figure 2-33

SPECIAL TECHNIQUES: WIRING CONFIGURATIONS

Many methods have been described for internal wire fixation of mandibular fractures. The wiring configuration that provides the greatest stabilization in any given situation is dictated by the plane of the fracture and the degree of comminution.

In the preceding example, the plane of the fracture is approximately perpendicular to the lateral and medial cortices of the bone and courses obliquely from inferior to superior. In such cases, one or two internal fixation wires, either one of which crosses the fracture at a right angle, usually provides good stability (Figure 2-33).

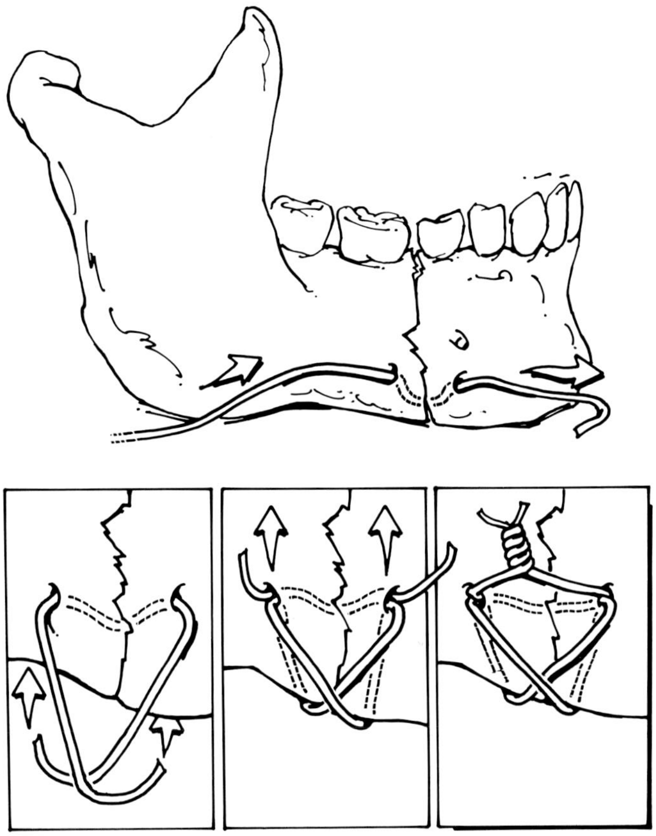

Figure 2-34

Fractures that course perpendicular to the lateral and medial cortical bone and are perpendicular to the inferior and superior borders of the mandible are in effect a "butt joint" and are best stabilized with an Obwegeser-type wiring technique when an internal wire is used (Figure 2-34).

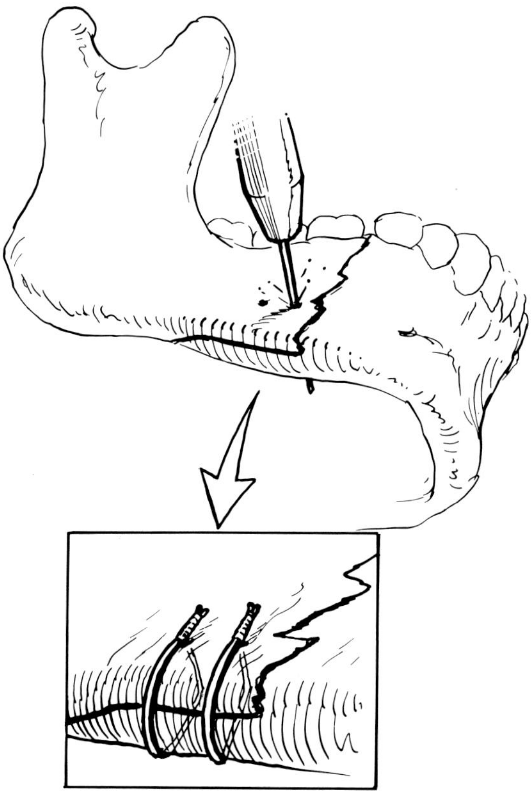

Figure 2-35

Fractures that course obliquely through the mandible in a sagittal fashion are best stabilized with two or more lag wires when an internal wire is used (Figure 2-35).

ECCENTRIC DYNAMIC COMPRESSION PLATES

The purpose of the eccentric dynamic compression plate is to provide compressive forces that are distributed over the entire surface of the fracture. This system is best suited for butt joint types of mandibular fractures.

Reduction compression pliers are applied to the inferior border of the mandible (Figure 2-36). As the pliers are closed, the inferior portion of the fracture is compressed. The lateral compression rollers set against the inferior border of the mandible cause the fragments to rotate about the inferior border, thereby reducing the superior border.

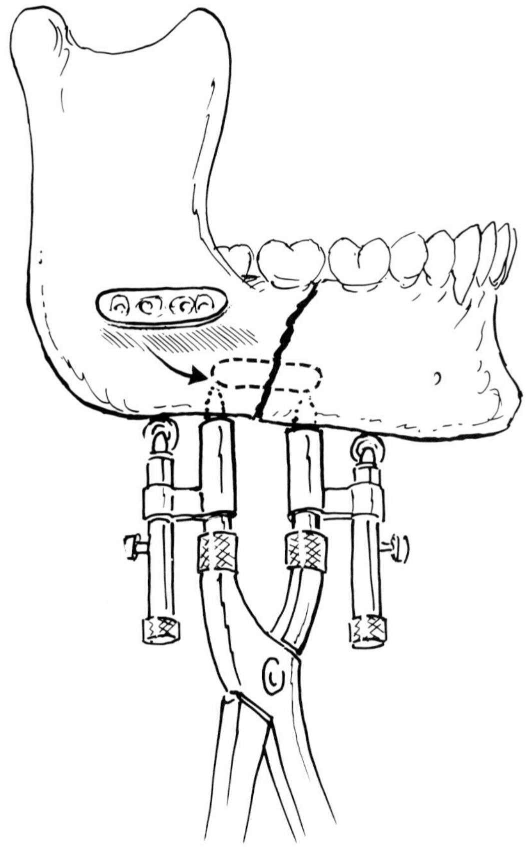

Figure 2-36

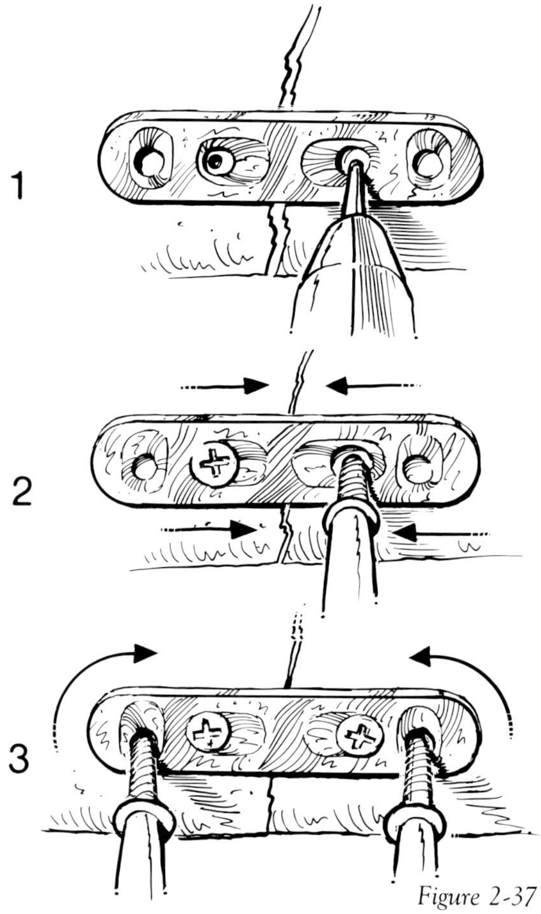

Figure 2-37

Holes are drilled and the innermost screws compress the inferior border as they are tightened in the eccentrically beveled holes of the plate (Figure 2-37). The outer screws are tightened, and the superior border is compressed as the fragments are forced to rotate about the first set of screws.

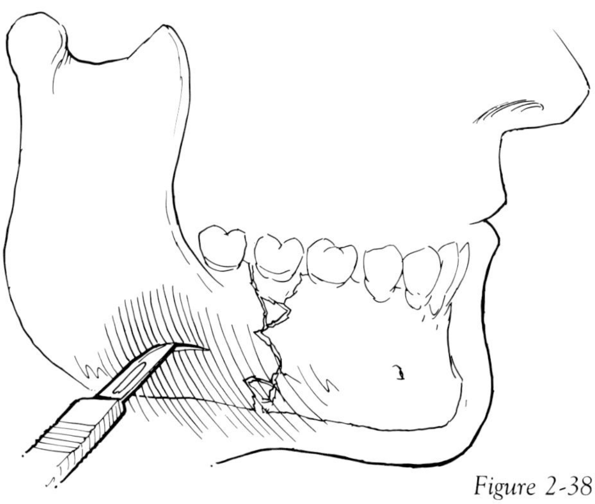
Figure 2-38

MORRIS EXTERNAL BIPHASE SPLINT

The external biphase splint is an invaluable adjunct in the management of injuries of the mandible involving avulsion of bone. It is also an excellent method for stabilization of unstable and grossly comminuted mandibular fractures and for stabilization of certain fractures of the edentulous mandible.

The face is prepared in the usual manner and draped so as to expose the entire lower face. The inferior border of the mandible is palpated and a skin incision approximately 1 cm in length is made 0.5–1 cm above and parallel to the inferior border of the mandible and approximately 1.5 cm from the fracture in the posterior fragment (Figure 2-38).

Blunt dissection to bone with a mosquito hemostat exposes the mandible (Figure 2-39).

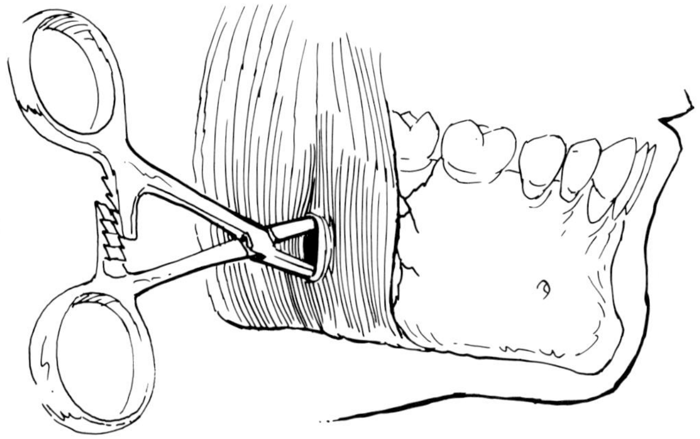

Figure 2-39

A 5/64-inch drill mounted in a Bunnell handpiece is inserted through the drill guide and used to penetrate both the lateral and medial cortices (Figure 2-40).

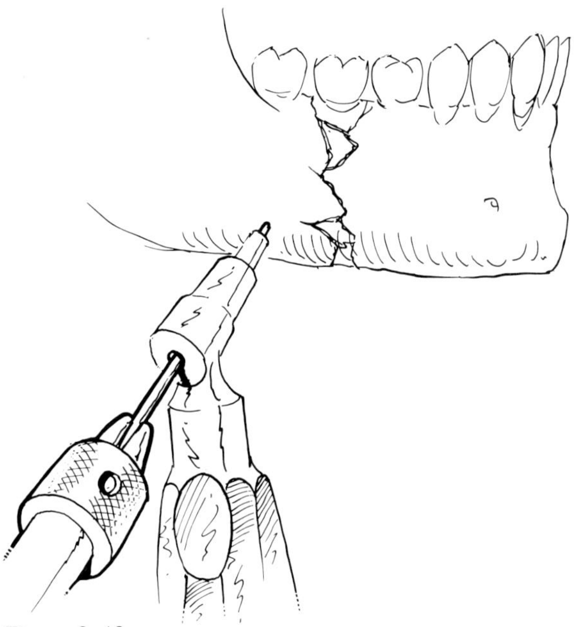

Figure 2-40

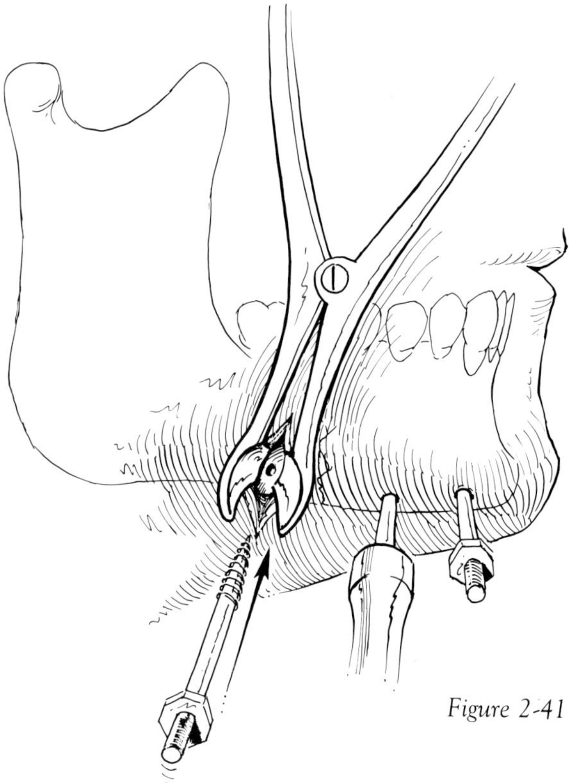

Figure 2-41

The drill hole in the bone is exposed with a small nasal speculum, and a pin is screwed into the bone with finger pressure and tightened with the pin wrench (Figure 2-41). Generally only one pin is necessary in the posterior fragment since the condyle seated in the glenoid fossa stabilizes the opposite end of this fragment. Two pins are placed in the anterior fragment. The pins are placed 3 cm apart and no closer than 1.5 cm to the fracture.

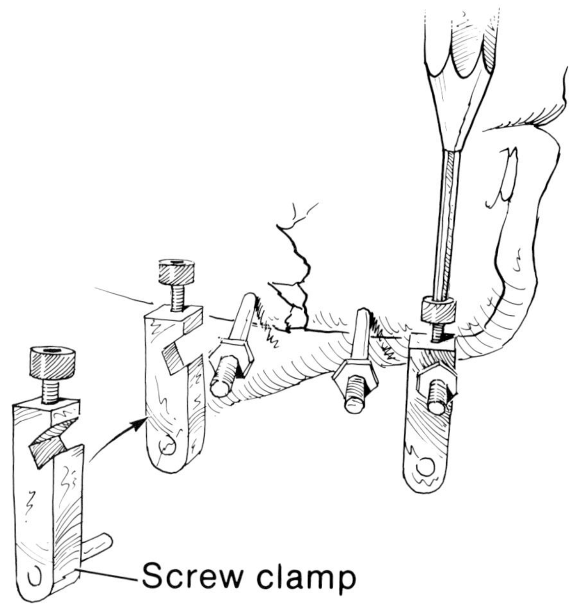

Figure 2-42

Screw clamps are placed immediately below the hexagonal table and tightened with the Allen wrench (Figure 2-42). One clamp is applied to the pin in the posterior fragment, and another clamp is applied to either pin in the anterior fragment.

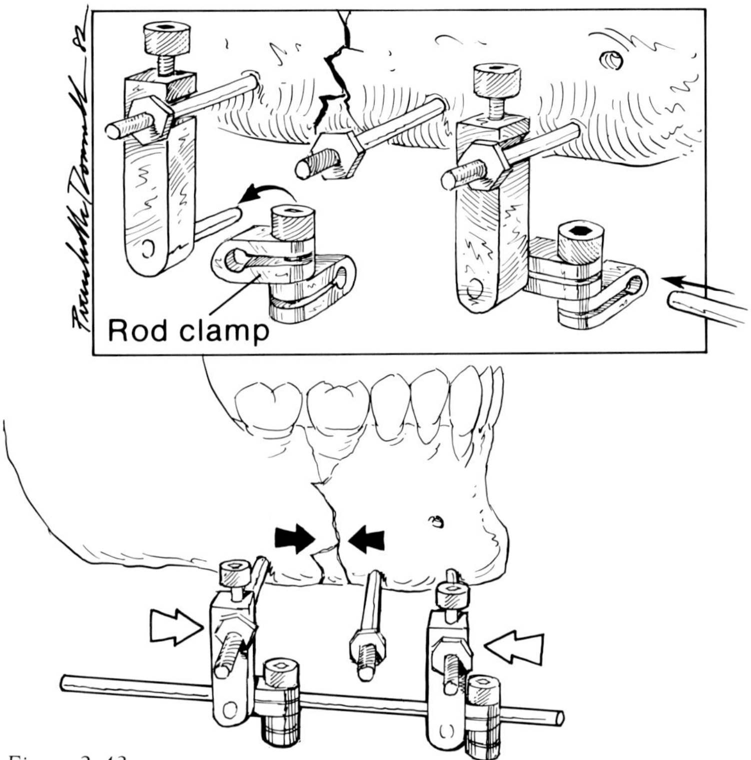

Figure 2-43

Rod clamps are placed onto the screw clamps, and the connector rod is passed through the rod clamps (Figure 2-43). The mandibular fragments are then brought into proper alignment, and the rod clamps are tightened with the Allen wrench, thereby stabilizing the fracture fragments.

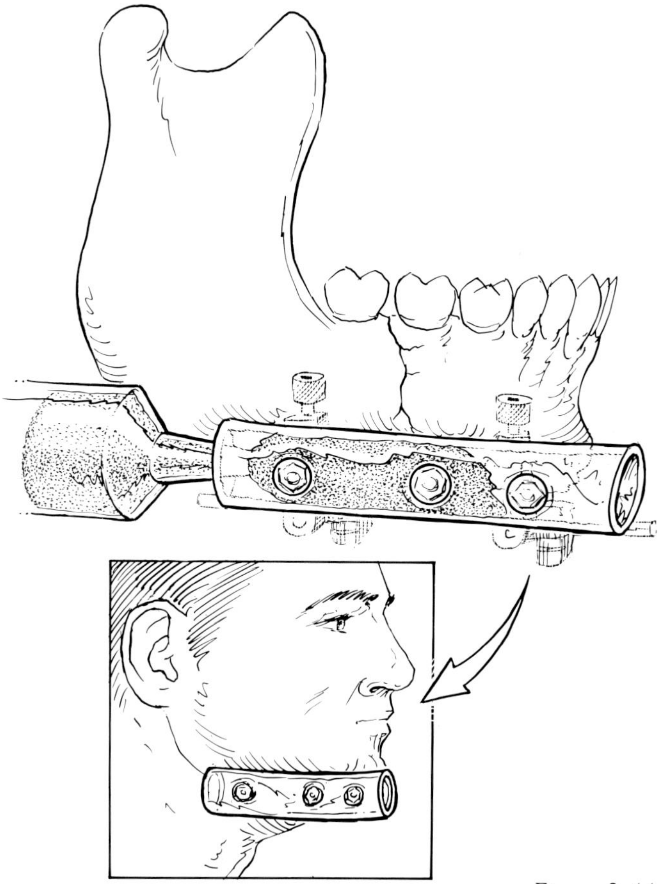

Figure 2-44

A 10-mm endotracheal tube is applied onto the terminal portion of the pins above the hexagonal table and fixed with the lock nuts (Figure 2-44). The endotracheal tube is then filled with self-curing acrylic resin using a 60-ml catheter tip syringe. After the resin is hardened, the screw clamps, rod clamps, and connector rod are removed.

REFERENCES

1. Gans, B. J.: Atlas of Oral Surgery. Mosby, St. Louis, p. 145, 1972.
2. Gilmer, T. L.: Fractures. In: Oral Surgery, S. V. Mead (Ed.). Mosby, St. Louis, pp. 694–696, 1954.
3. Kazanjian, V. H. and Converse, J. M.: Surgical Treatment of Facial Fractures, Vol. 1. Williams & Wilkins, Baltimore, pp. 157–158, 1974.
4. Kruger, G. O.: Textbook of Oral Surgery. Mosby, St. Louis, pp. 320–321, 1968.
5. Morris, J. H.: Biphase Connector, External Skeletal Splint for Reduction and Fixation of Mandibular Fractures. *Oral Surg.*, 2:1382–1398, 1949.
6. Schmoker, R.: Exzentrisch Dynamische Kompressionsplatte sowie Kompressions-Zuggurtungsschiene, Kompressions-Zuggurtungsplatte und Repositions-Kompressionszange. Eine neve Technik der funktionsstabilen Unterkieferosteosynthese mit Kompression auf der Zugseite. Dissertation, Basel, 1973.

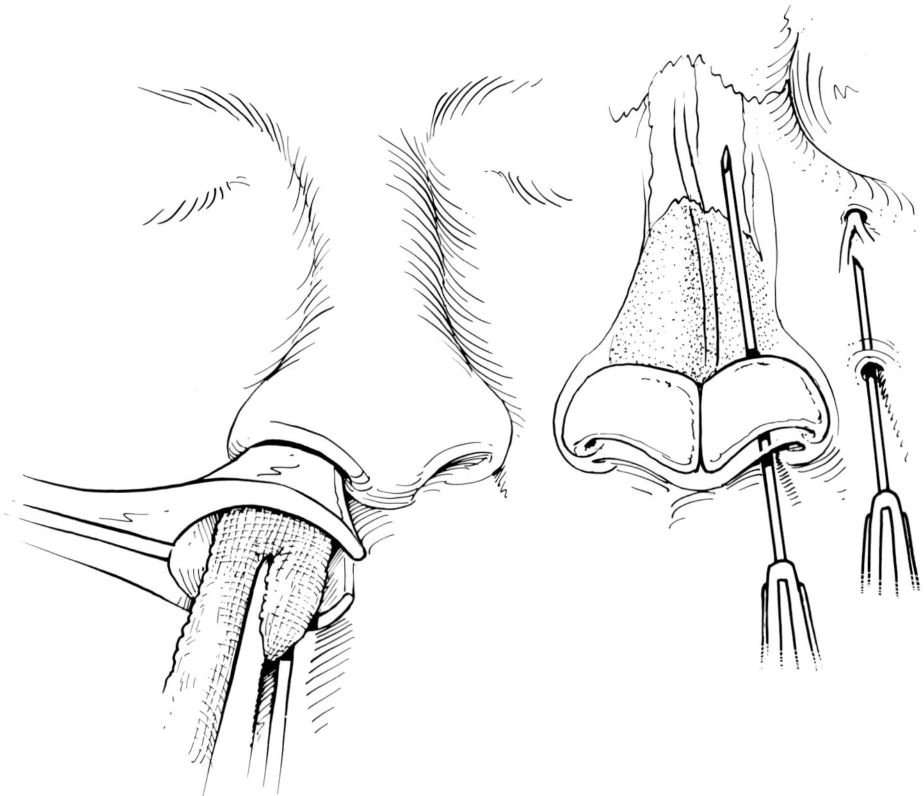

Figure 3-3

SEPTAL DISLOCATION

Anesthesia is obtained by placing a 12-inch length of cocaine-impregnated cotton gauze in both nostrils (Figure 3-3). Then 1% lidocaine with epinephrine 1:100,000 is infiltrated sparingly over the dorsum of the nose, in the area of the infraorbital foramina, and in the septal mucosa.

The Asche forceps are used to reposition the quadrilateral cartilage on the maxillary crest (Figure 3-4). Gentle dorsal pressure on the septal cartilage makes the reduction easier. Packing is left in both nostrils for approximately 5 days to maintain the reduction.

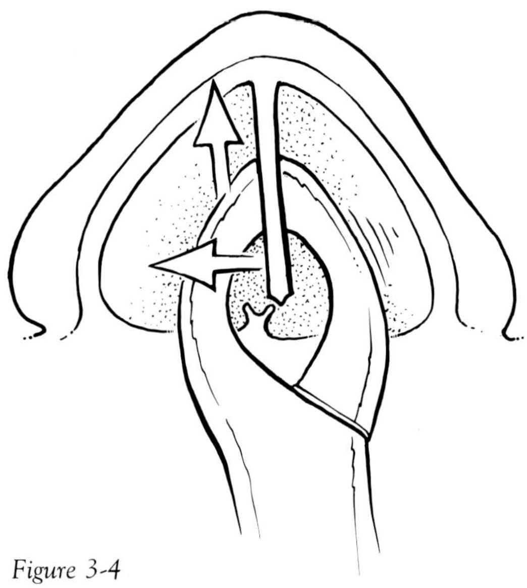

Figure 3-4

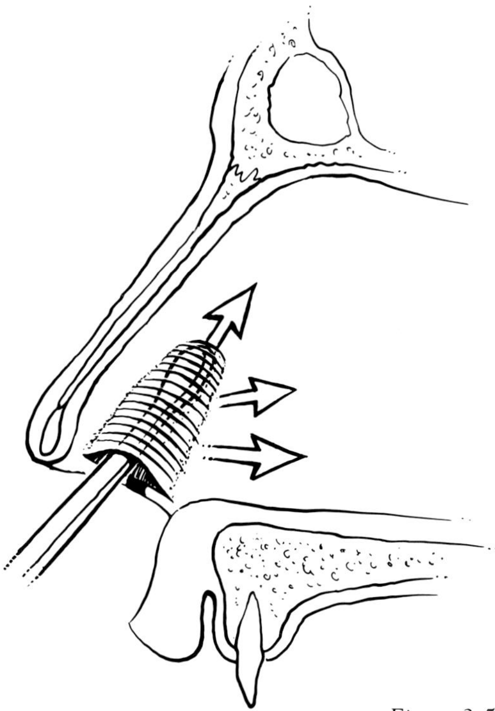

Figure 3-5

If closed reduction of the septal dislocation is not successful, then open reduction is indicated. A hemitransfixion incision is made and a mucoperichondrial flap is elevated on the side to which the septal cartilage is dislocated (Figure 3-5).

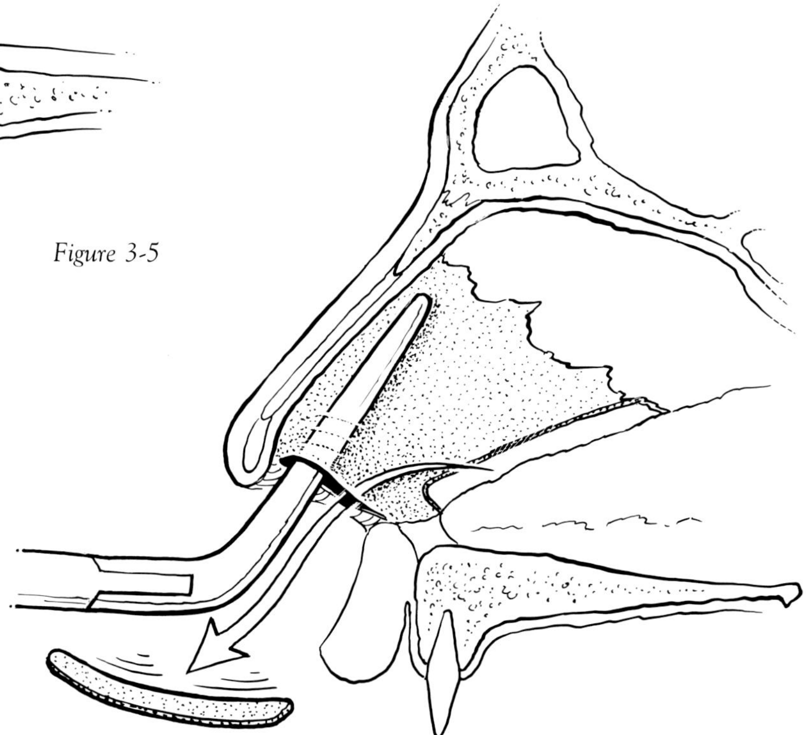

Figure 3-6

By direct manipulation, the septal cartilage is replaced on the maxillary crest (Figure 3-6). It may be necessary to excise a small portion of septal cartilage at the level of the maxillary crest in order to obtain a reduction. The hemitransfixion incision is closed with absorbable sutures, and packing is placed in the nose.

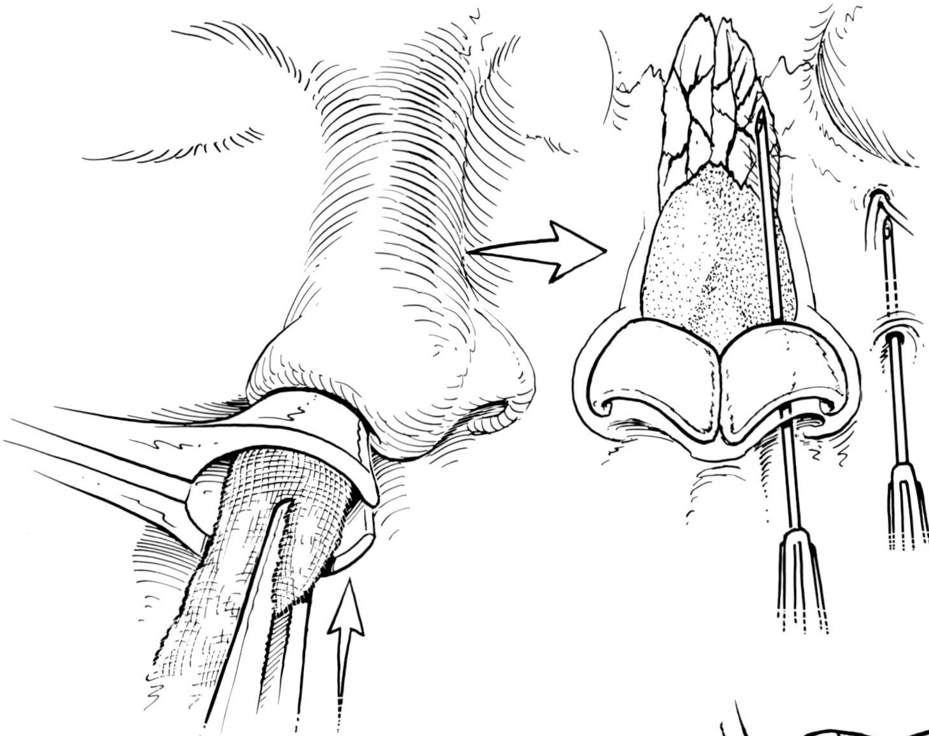

Figure 3-7

NASAL FRACTURE

CLOSED REDUCTION

Most nasal fractures can be reduced satisfactorily using a closed technique.

Anesthesia is obtained by placing cocaine-impregnated cotton gauze in both nostrils and infiltrating with 1% lidocaine with epinephrine 1:100,000 sparingly over the dorsum of the nose and in the area of the infraorbital foramina (Figure 3-7).

Frequently the nasal bones are displaced posteriorly in addition to being displaced laterally (Figure 3-8). Elevation can be accomplished by placing a scalpel handle or other elevator in the nasal cavity and elevating the fragments dorsally. Pressure applied from the lateral surface of the nose simultaneously provides a very nice reduction.

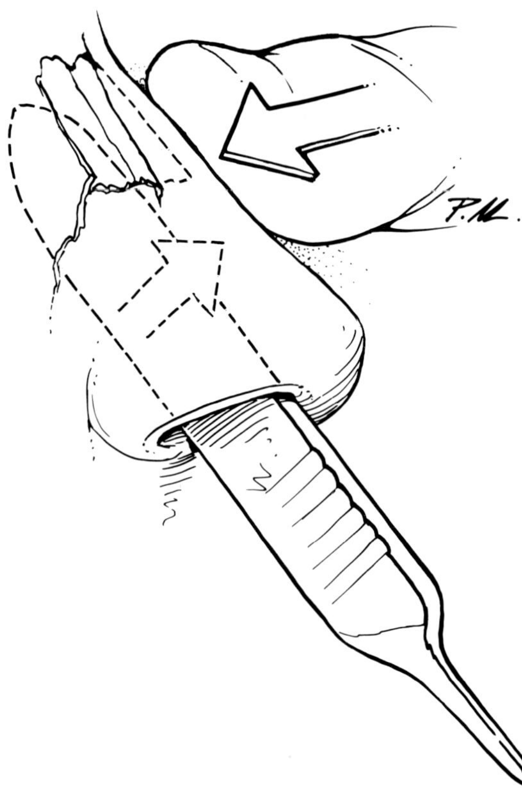

Figure 3-8

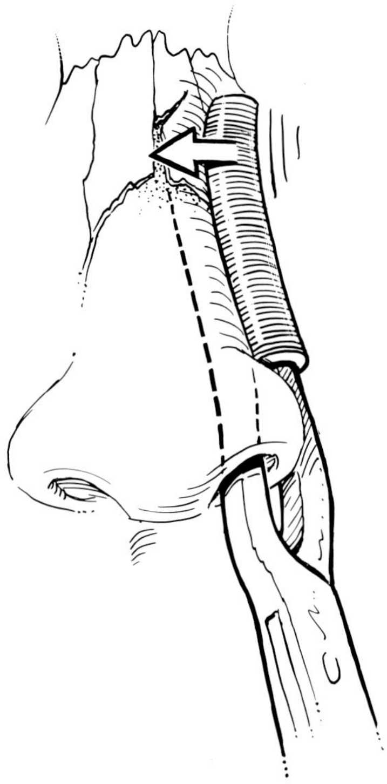

Figure 3-9

A variety of forceps can also be used to manipulate the nasal bones into position (Figure 3-9). The nasal cavity is lightly packed so as to maintain the reduction but not distort the nose.

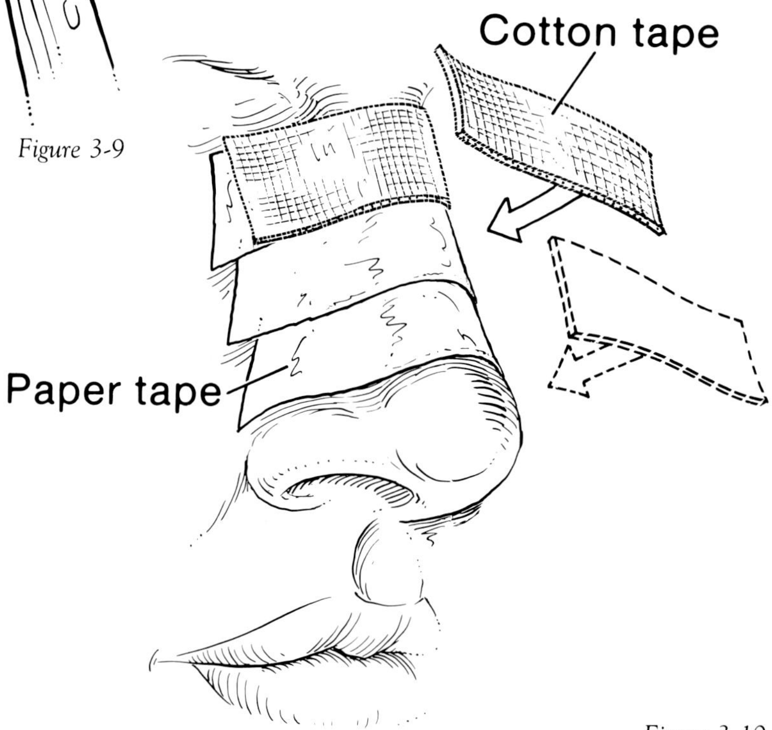

Figure 3-10

Benzoin is applied to the dorsum of the nose, followed by a layer of paper tape and then cotton adhesive tape (Figure 3-10).

Five layers of cast material are cut into the appropriately shaped splint and then moistened in warm water (Figure 3-11). The cast is applied to the cotton tape and molded to the proper position. The cast is removed 7 days later.

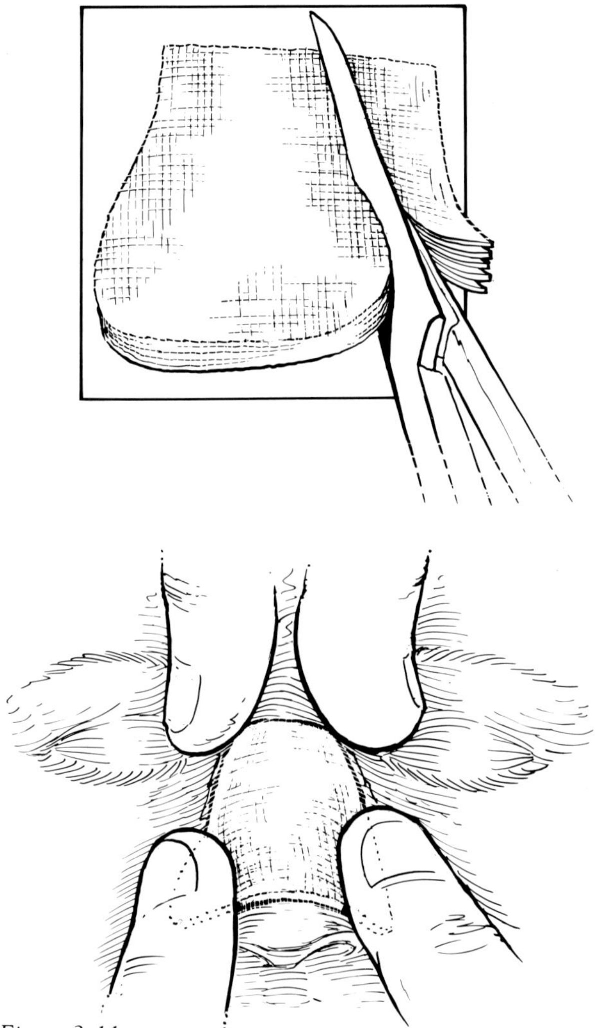

Figure 3-11

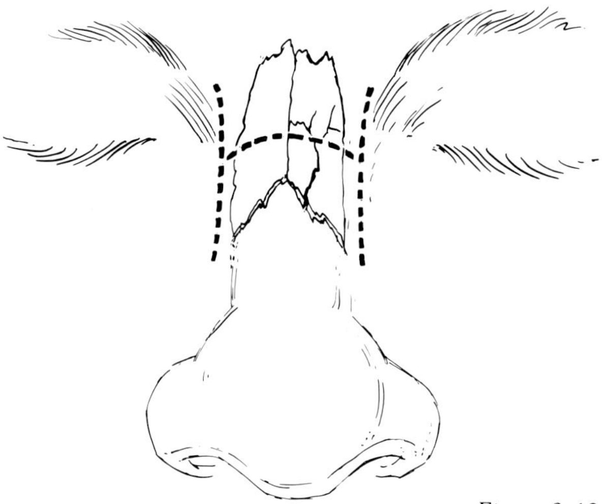

Figure 3-12

OPEN REDUCTION AND INTERNAL FIXATION

In certain severe nasal fractures it may be difficult to obtain and maintain reduction by the closed technique. In these unusual cases it may be necessary to perform an open reduction of the nasal bones.

Parallel incisions are made on both sides of the nose one-half the distance between the dorsum of the nose and the medial canthus (Figure 3-12). A connecting incision is made over the root of the nose, and the skin flaps are elevated to expose the nasal bones.

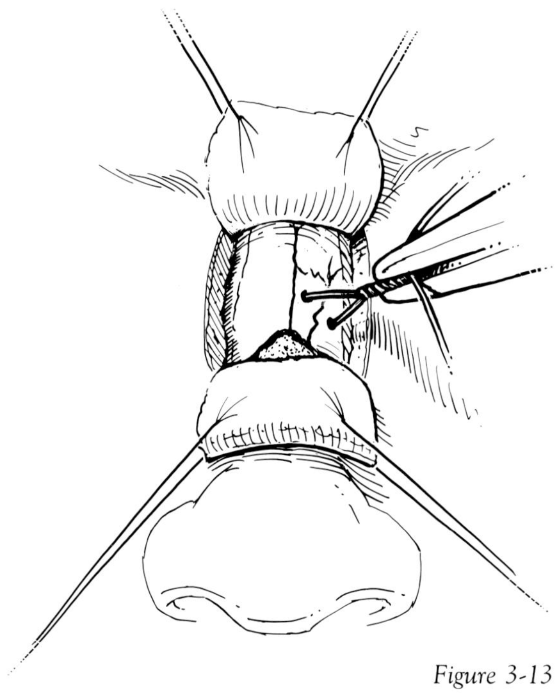

Figure 3-13

The fracture fragments are reduced and wired in position with stainless steel wire (Figure 3-13). It may be necessary to obtain this fixation only on the larger fragments, which will then support the smaller, more comminuted fragments.

Small absorbable sutures are placed in the subcutaneous tissue (Figure 3-14). Gillies' corner sutures are used to approximate the wound, and the remainder of the incision is closed in a subcuticular fashion.

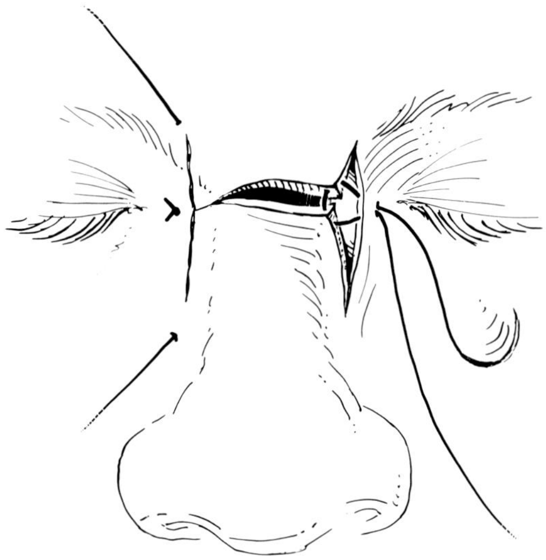

Figure 3-14

REFERENCES

1. Converse, J. M. and Hogan, V. M.: Open-Sky Approach for Reduction of Naso-orbital Fractures: Case Report. *Plast. Reconstr. Surg.*, 46:396–398, 1970.

4

Fractures of the Frontal Sinus

In addition to the cosmetic deformity, frontal sinus fractures can expose the patient to a variety of serious sequelae. The relationship of the brain, frontal sinus, and nasofrontal ostium is depicted in Figure 4-1. If a fracture has occurred through the nasofrontal ostium then inadequate drainage of mucous may occur, leading to the formation of a mucocele. Fractures of the posterior wall of the sinus create a direct communication between the frontal sinus and the intracranial cavity, which may lead to meningitis, brain abscess, and other intracranial complications.

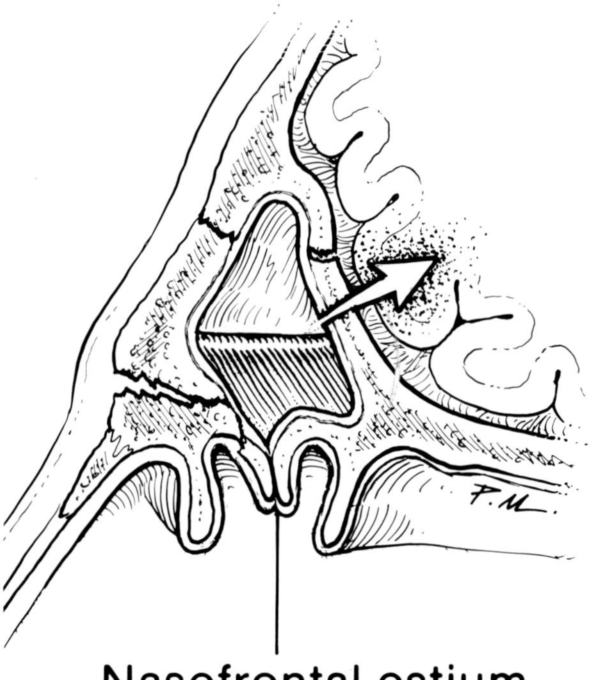

Figure 4-1

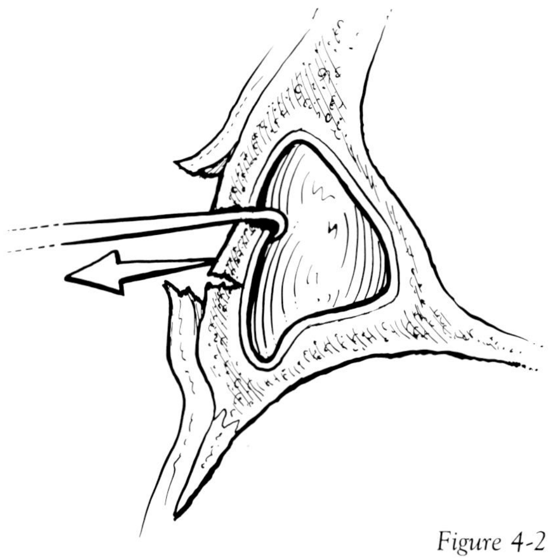

Figure 4-2

FRACTURES OF THE ANTERIOR WALL

If only the anterior wall of the frontal sinus is fractured, then reduction without obliteration of the frontal sinus is performed.

There is frequently a skin laceration overlying the area of the frontal sinus fracture (Figure 4-2); if not, exposure can be obtained through the coronal or brow incisions. Skin hooks are placed underneath the fracture fragments, which are elevated into position.

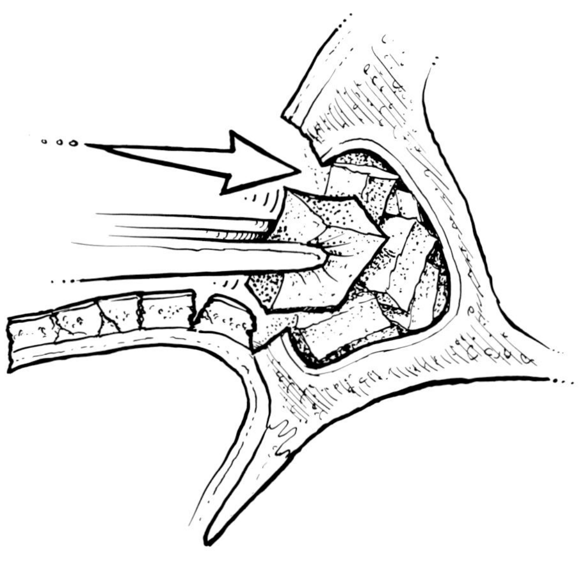

Figure 4-3

If the reduction cannot be maintained, an exploration of the frontal sinus through an osteoplastic flap and placement of Gelfoam in the sinus to support the fracture fragments may be indicated (Figure 4-3).

FRACTURES INVOLVING THE NASOFRONTAL OSTIA AND POSTERIOR WALL

If the posterior wall or nasofrontal ostia are involved, then the frontal sinus should be obliterated to prevent future complications.

Two incisions are available for exploration of the frontal sinus (Figure 4-4). The coronal incision is probably the most cosmetically pleasing except in the balding patient. It also provides excellent exposure for a craniotomy, which may be required in conjunction with frontal sinus exploration and obliteration. The brow incision is useful in smaller frontal sinuses; however, in a patient with extremely large frontal sinuses the exposure is limited. In the trauma patient there is frequently a laceration in the area of the brow that can be easily incorporated into a brow incision.

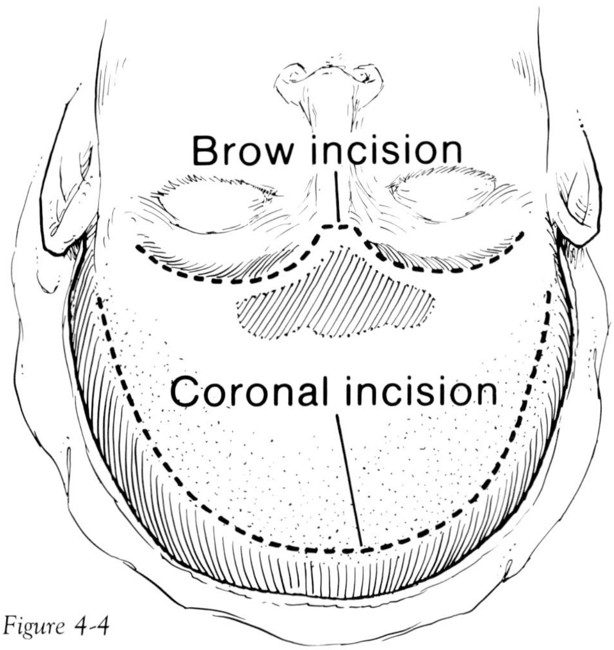

Figure 4-4

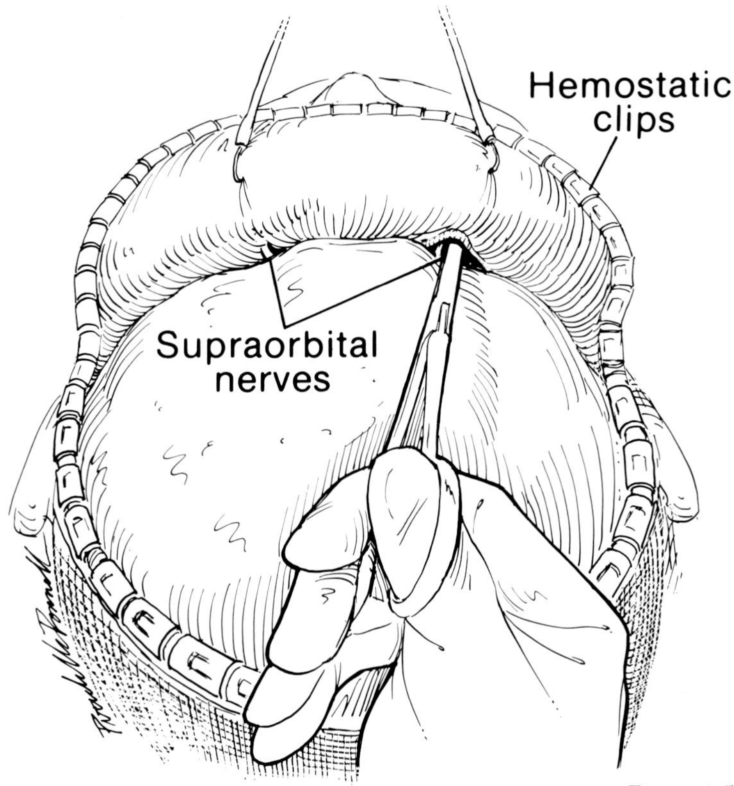

Figure 4-5

The flap is elevated in a plane just superficial to the periosteum, which should remain intact (Figure 4-5). If the coronal incision is used, blunt dissection in the area of the supraorbital nerves helps identify and preserve these nerves. The flap is then retracted using "fish-hooks" on elastics.

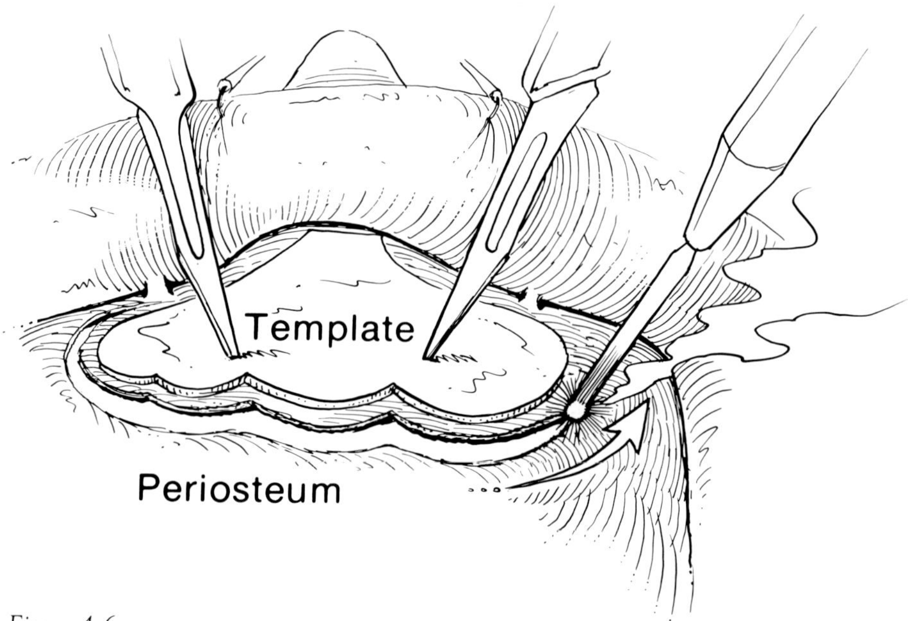

Figure 4-6

A template made from a 6-foot Caldwell view of the skull is positioned over the frontal bone and held in place by scalpels with No. 11 blades (Figure 4-6). The Bovie cautery is used to incise the periosteum superiorly and laterally.

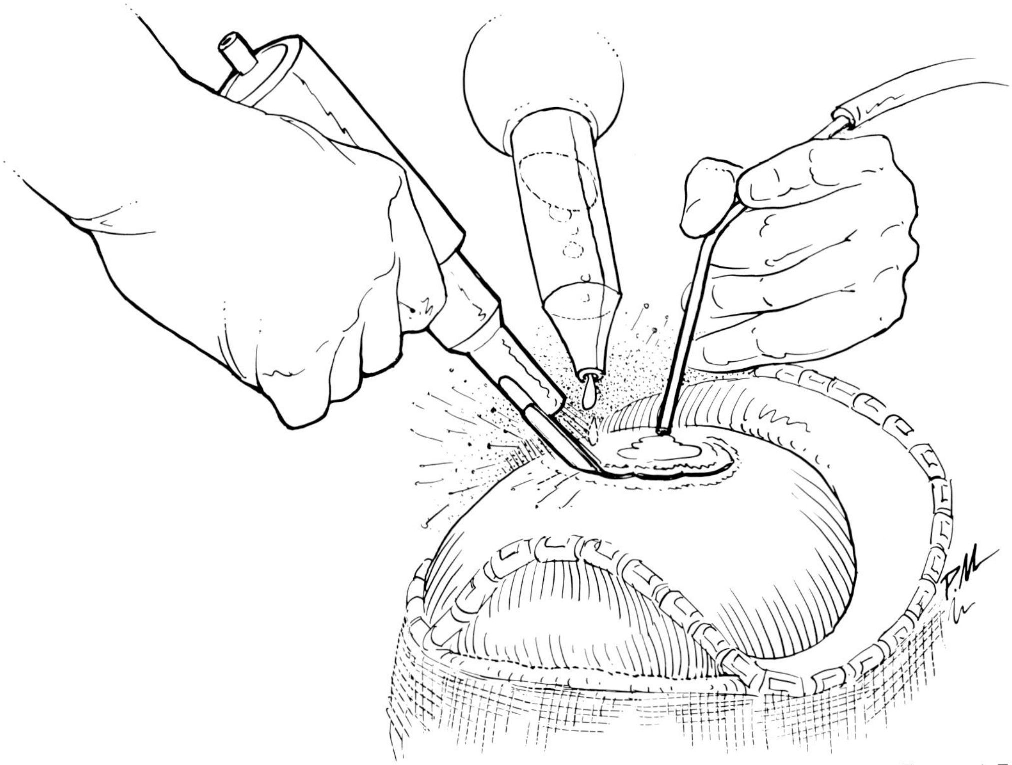

Figure 4-7

The periosteum is elevated for a short distance toward the floor of the frontal sinus, and then the bone is cut with the oscillating saw (Figure 4-7). Care is taken not to injure the periosteum with the saw. The bone cuts must be beveled in order to provide support for the bone flap when it is replaced.

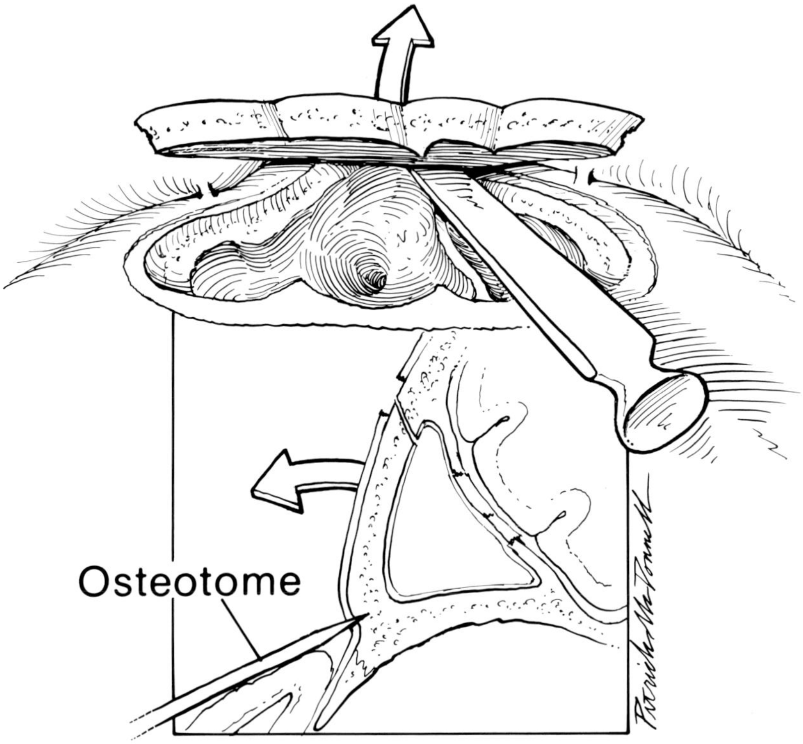

Figure 4-8

Small osteotomes are used to elevate the bone flap (Figure 4-8). The osteotomes can be used to transect the septa of the frontal sinus if elevation of the flap is difficult. Occasionally, an inferior osteotomy is necessary to facilitate elevation of the flap.

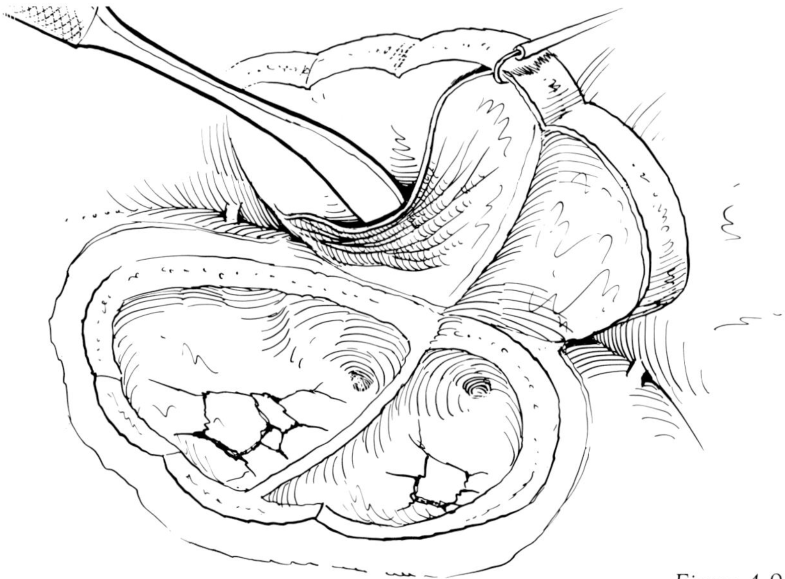

Figure 4-9

The bone flap is retracted inferiorly (Figure 4-9). Care must be taken to maintain the integrity of the periosteum and bone, particularly when the anterior wall of the frontal sinus is comminuted. The mucosa of the frontal sinus is carefully removed.

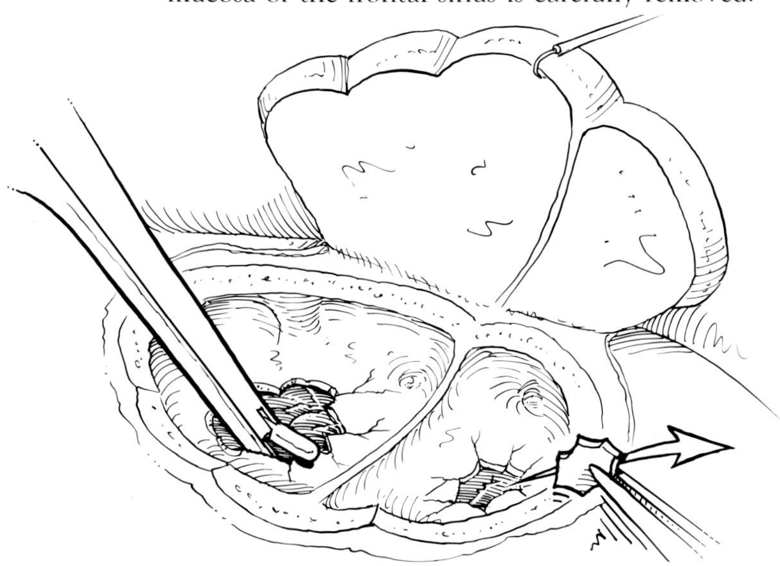

Figure 4-10

Posterior wall bone fragments are carefully dissected free of the dura and removed (Figure 4-10). The edges of the fractures are also carefully rongeured to expose the underlying dura.

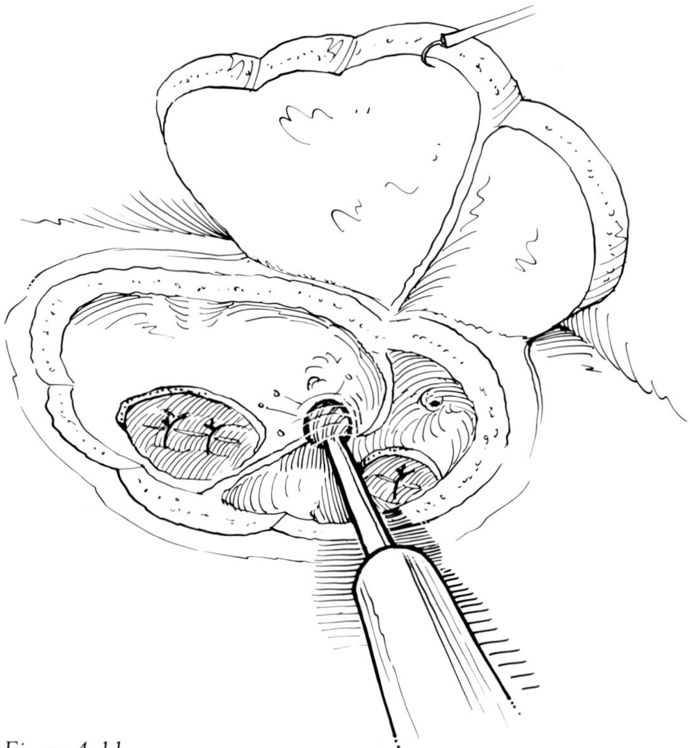

Figure 4-11

If a dural laceration is present it should be closed using 4-0 silk sutures (Figure 4-11). Any remaining mucosa is removed with an elevator and a cutting bur is used to drill the bony septa flush with the walls of the frontal sinus.

A diamond bur and the operating microscope are used to drill carefully the walls of the frontal sinus to remove any residual mucosa (Figure 4-12).

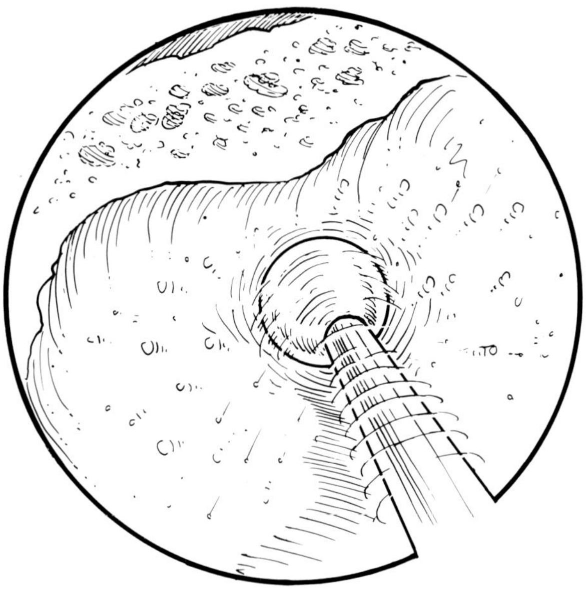

Figure 4-12

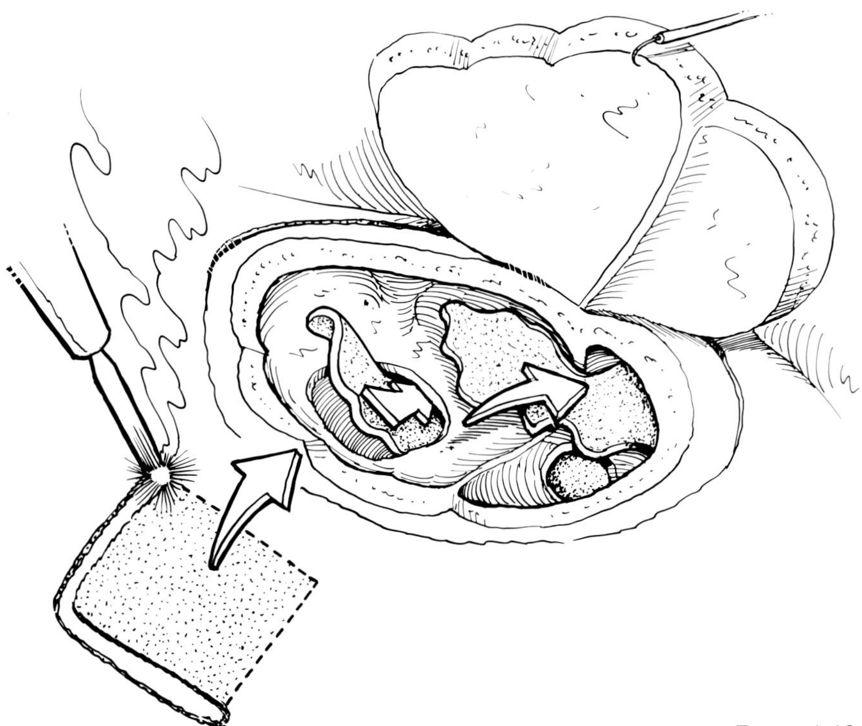

Figure 4-13

A piece of pericranium is placed over the naso-frontal ostia and the dural repairs (Figure 4-13).

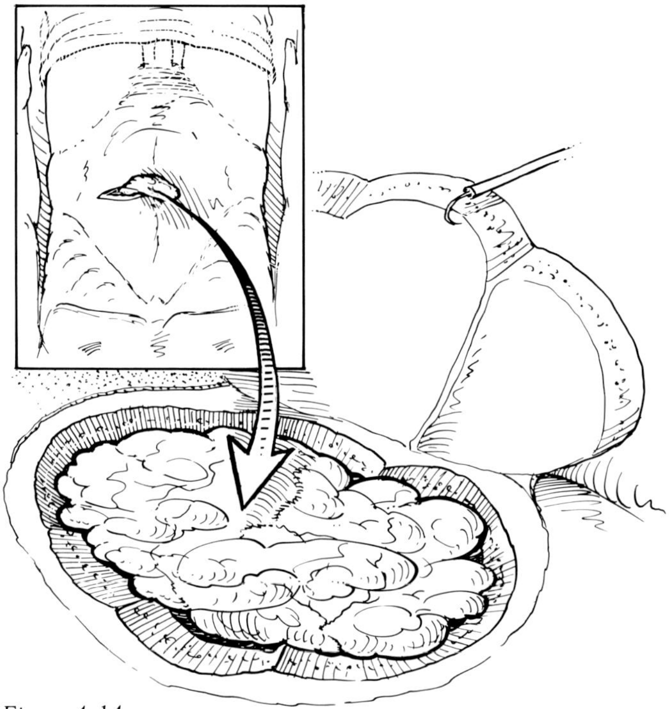

Figure 4-14

Another member of the surgical team has removed fat from a left-sided abdominal incision. Right-sided incisions are avoided because if the patient were to have appendicitis in the future, an unsuspecting physician might think that the patient already had had an appendectomy. As much as possible, the fat is placed in the frontal sinus in one piece (Figure 4-14). The bone flap is then reflected back into its position, and the periosteum is closed with absorbable sutures.

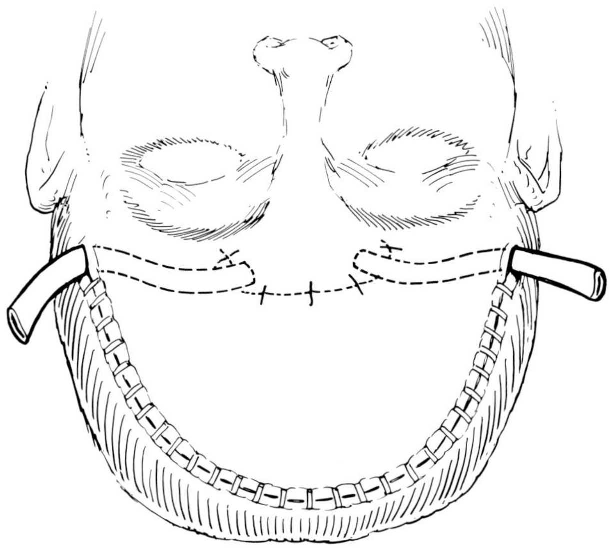

Figure 4-15

Penrose drains are placed over the frontal bone, the skin flap is replaced, and the incision is closed (Figure 4-15).

REFERENCES

1. Hybels, R. L.: Posterior Table Fractures of the Frontal Sinus: II. Clinical Aspects. *Laryngoscope,* 87:1740–1745, 1977.
2. Hybels, R. L. and Newman, M. H.: Posterior Table Fractures of the Frontal Sinus: I. An Experimental Study. *Laryngoscope,* 87:171–179, 1977.
3. Newman, M. H. and Travis, L. W.: Frontal Sinus Fractures. *Laryngoscope,* 83:1281–1292, 1973.

5

Fractures of the Zygoma

CLOSED REDUCTION

A towel clip can be used to grasp the malar bone and achieve satisfactory reduction (Figure 5-1). In selected cases the reduction can be maintained without any further manipulation.

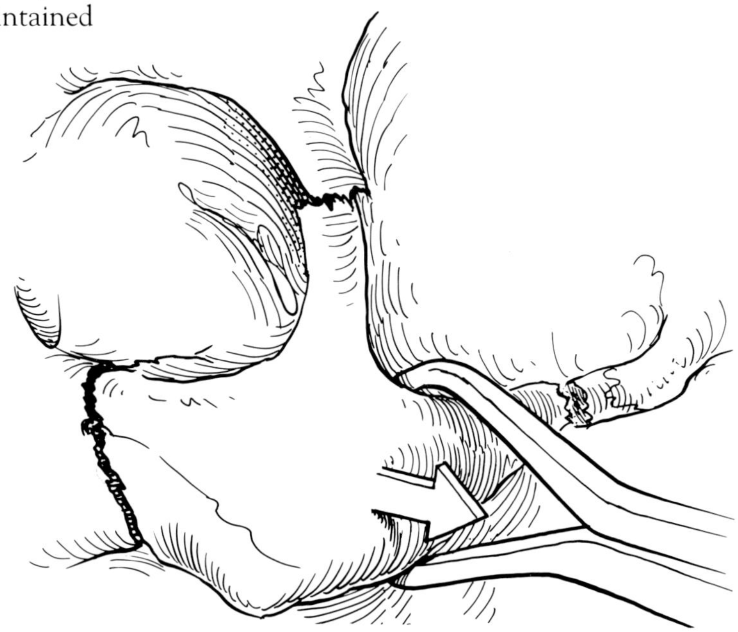

Figure 5-1

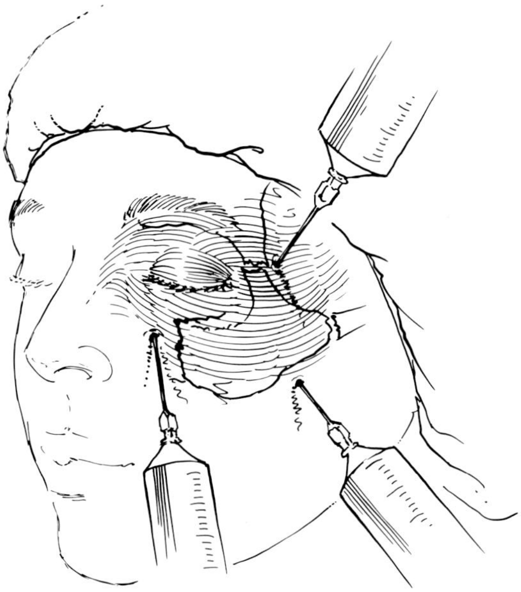

Figure 5-2

OPEN REDUCTION AND INTERNAL FIXATION

PERCUTANEOUS TECHNIQUE

The patient is placed on the operating table in a supine position with the back of the table somewhat elevated to reduce bleeding. Prior to preparation of the patient's face, 1% lidocaine with epinephrine 1:100,000 is infiltrated into the area of the initial incisions (Figure 5-2). The entire face is prepared so that the normal side can be compared to the injured side.

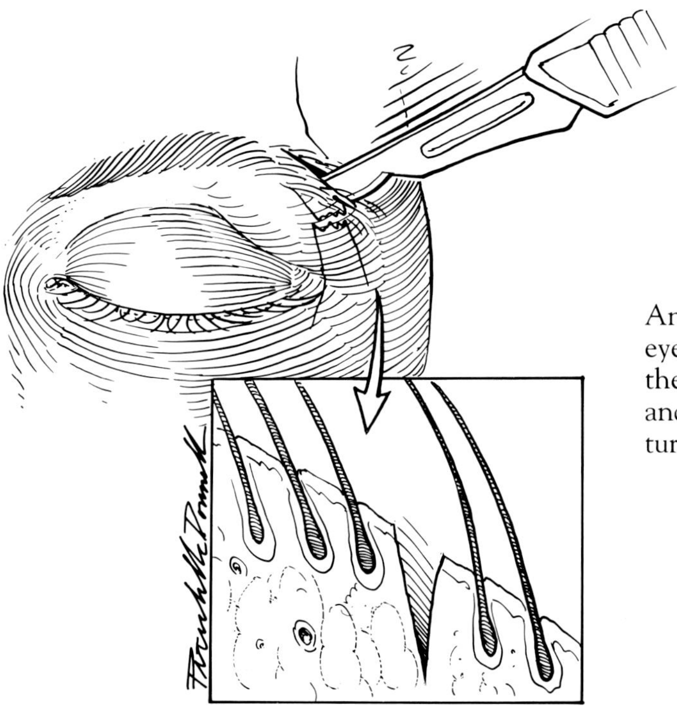

Figure 5-3

An incision is made in the lateral portion of the eyebrow; the incision is carefully beveled to parallel the shafts of the eyebrow hairs (Figure 5-3). Sharp and blunt dissection are used to identify the fracture in the area of the zygomaticofrontal suture.

Soft tissue is carefully curetted from the fracture line (Figure 5-4).

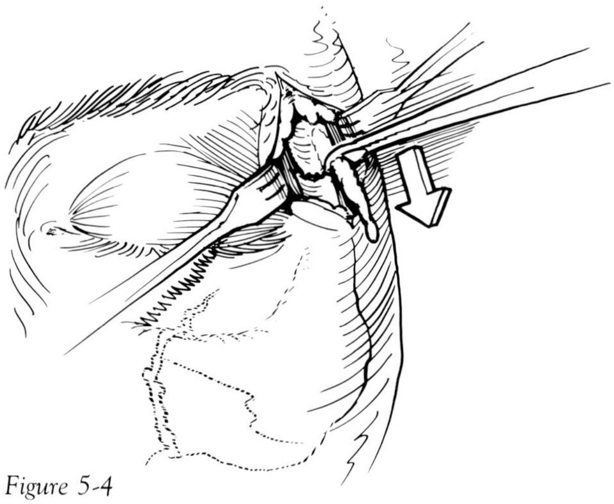

Figure 5-4

Two alternative incisions can be used for the infraorbital rim (Figure 5-5). An infraciliary incision, although cosmetically pleasing, may give rise to excessive edema of the eyelid. The author prefers making the incision in an existing skin crease more inferiorly on the eyelid, which provides a more direct approach to the infraorbital rim.

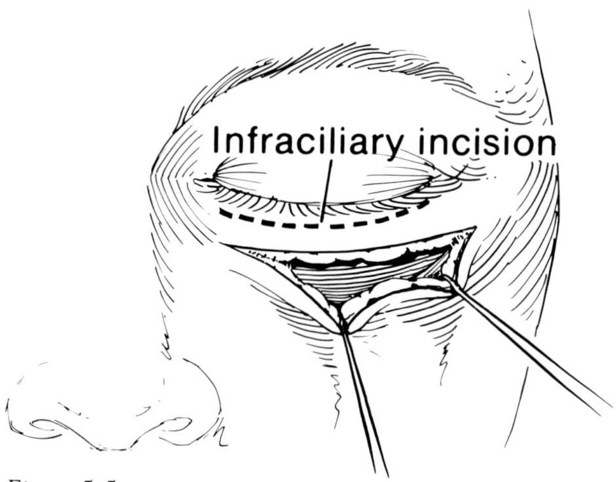

Figure 5-5

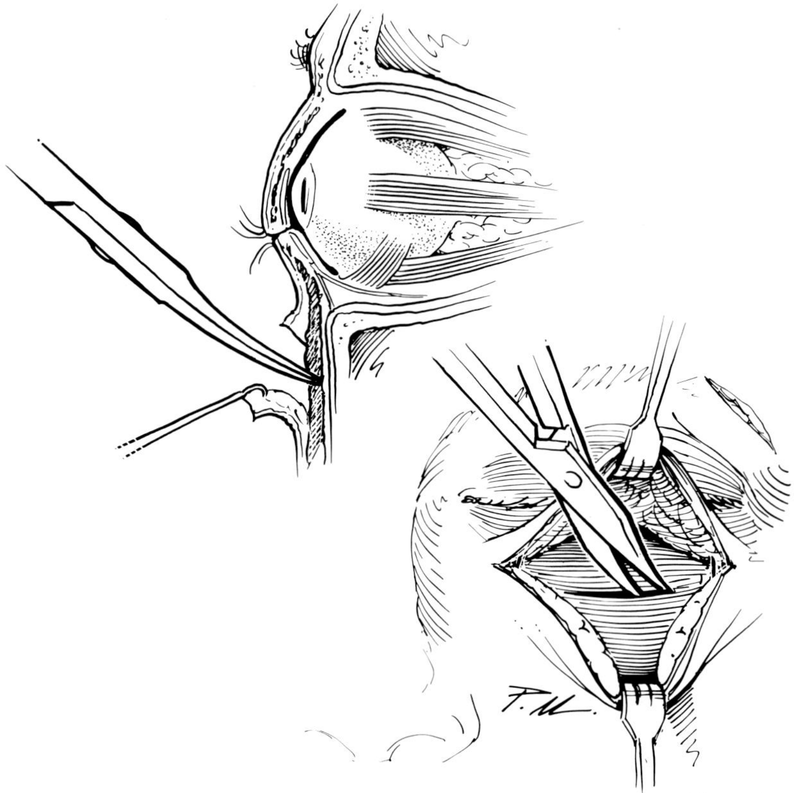

Figure 5-6

A small skin flap is elevated inferiorly and the orbicularis oculi muscle is separated longitudinally to expose the infraorbital rim (Figure 5-6). Placing the skin and muscle incisions at different levels provides a better cosmetic result.

The periosteum along the infraorbital rim is incised and carefully elevated along the orbital floor (Figure 5-7). The infraorbital fracture should be apparent at this time.

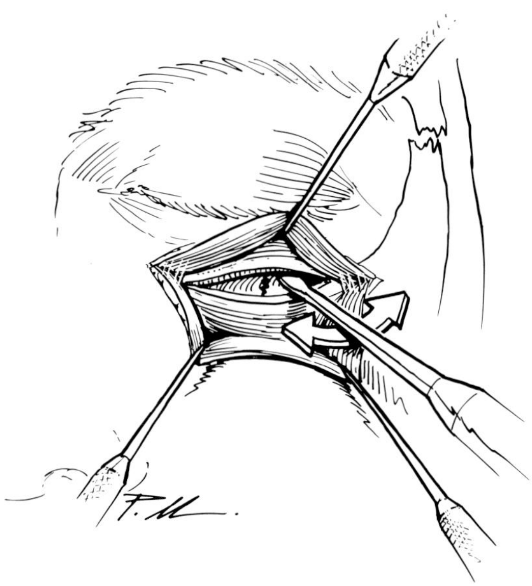

Figure 5-7

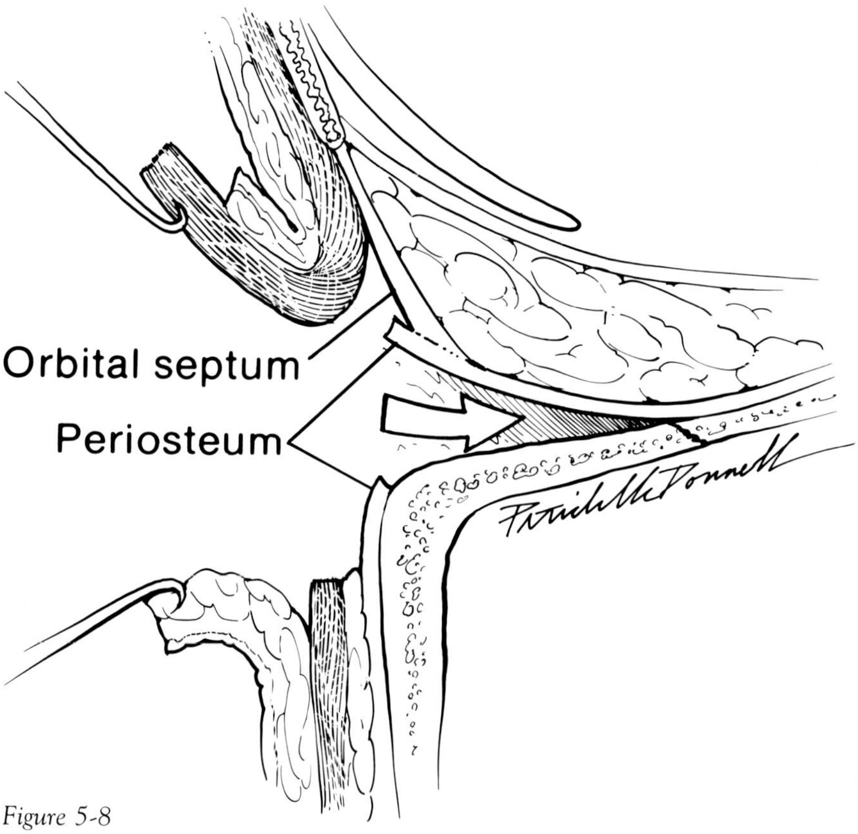

Figure 5-8

Periosteal elevators are used to elevate the periosteum off the orbital floor (Figure 5-8). Extreme care is taken not to injure the periosteum, as this would allow oribtal fat to herniate into the area, making the dissection more difficult.

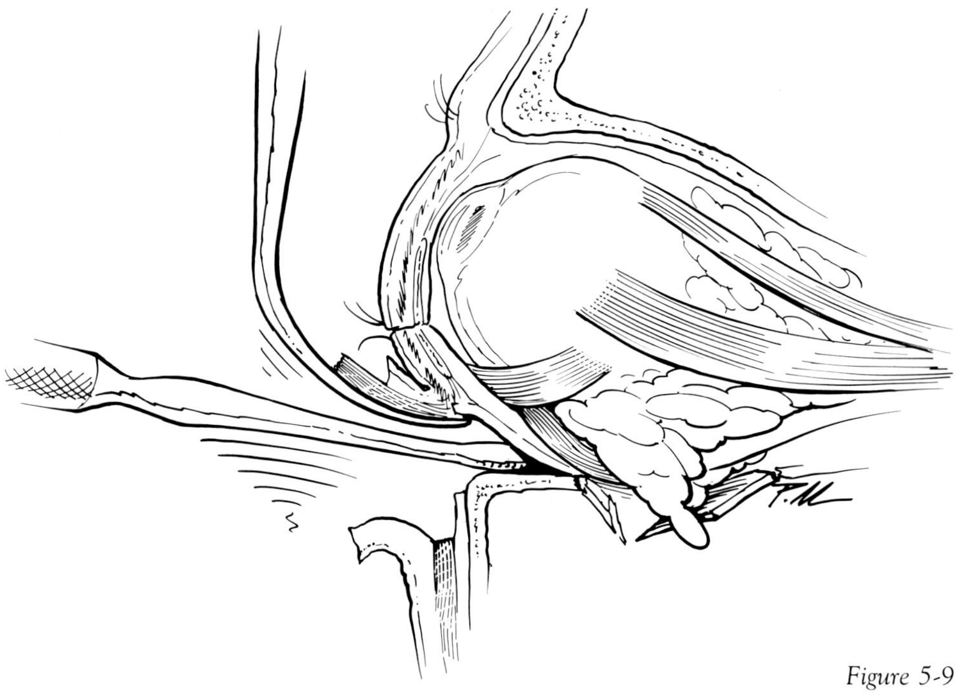

Figure 5-9

Orbital retractors are used carefully to retract the orbital contents, and the orbital floor is examined (Figure 5-9). Any entrapped orbital contents, such as fat or inferior rectus muscle, are carefully teased from the fracture line and returned to their normal position. It may be necessary to retract the malar bone in order to open the fracture and make freeing of the entrapped contents easier.

The malar bone is manipulated with bone hooks or bone clamps into its normal position (Figure 5-10). In some cases transantral manipulation (described later) may be very helpful in reducing the fracture.

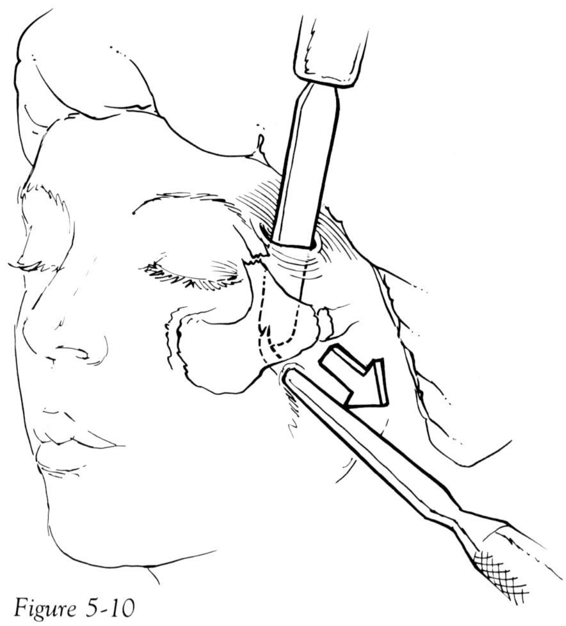

Figure 5-10

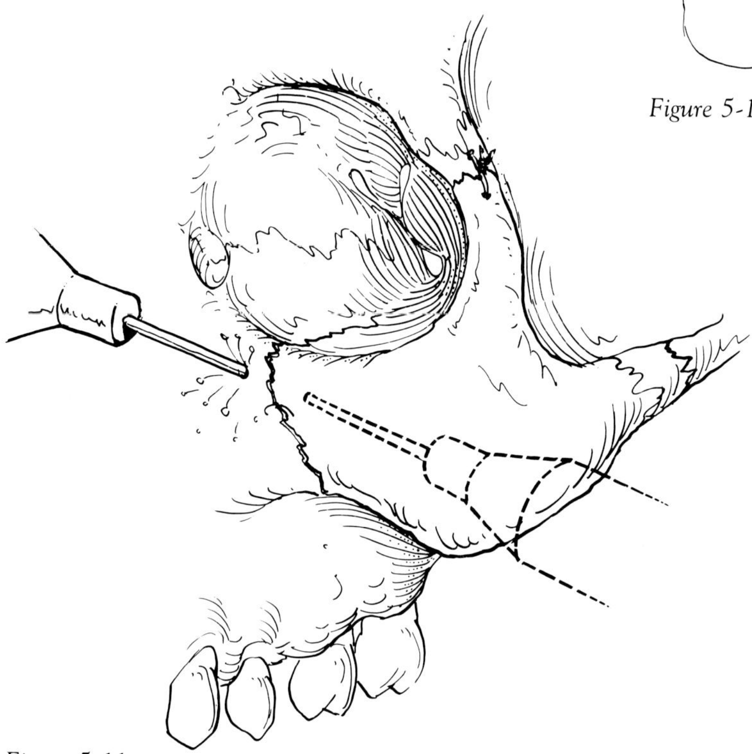

Figure 5-11

Holes are drilled on both sides of the zygomaticofrontal and the infraorbital rim fractures (Figure 5-11). Wires are passed.

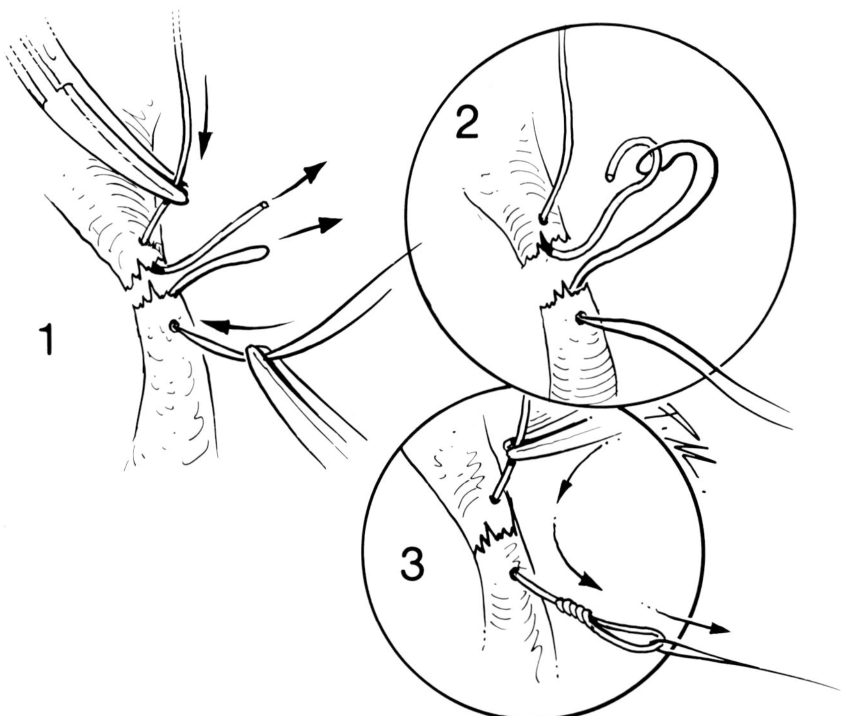

Figure 5-12

A wire bent on itself can be used as a wire passer (Figure 5-12).

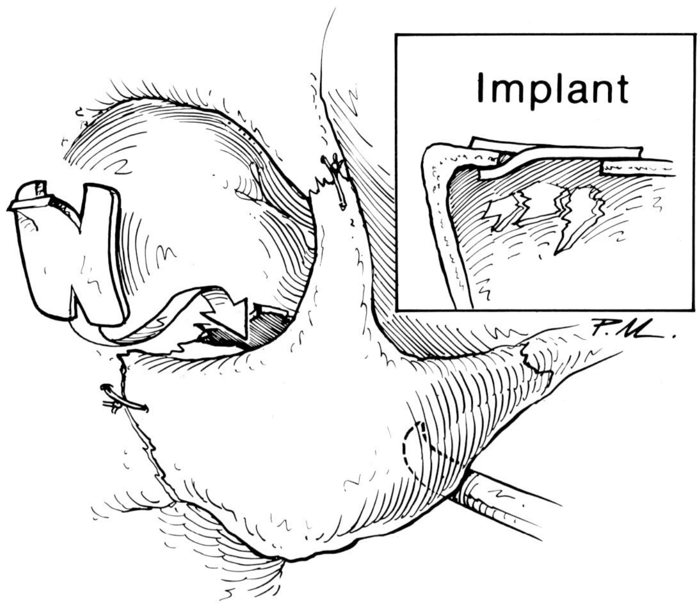

Figure 5-13

With the fracture held in place, the wires are carefully tightened (Figure 5-13). Care is taken not to pull them through the fragile bone, particularly the infraorbital rim. The orbital floor should be reexamined following reduction; if a significant dehiscence exists then an implant may be indicated. The author's preference is to use Gelfilm or Teflon. A flap can be cut in the implant so that it maintains its position.

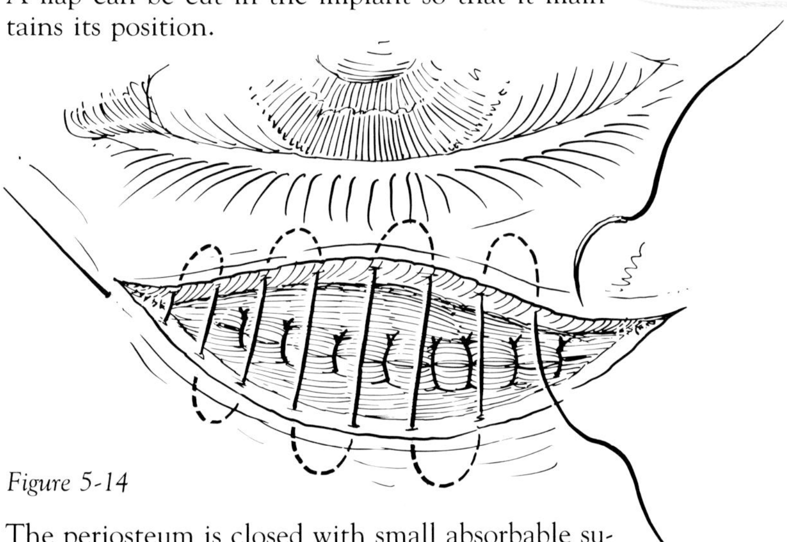

Figure 5-14

The periosteum is closed with small absorbable sutures, and the skin incisions are closed in a subcuticular fashion (Figure 5-14).

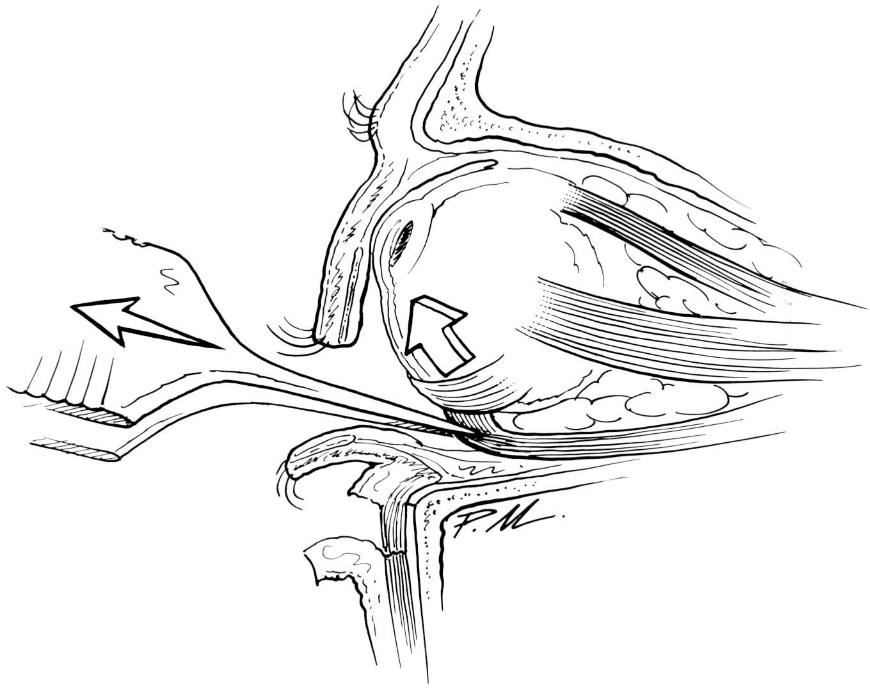

Figure 5-15

Forced duction testing should be performed to make sure that no orbital contents were entrapped during reduction of the fracture (Figure 5-15).

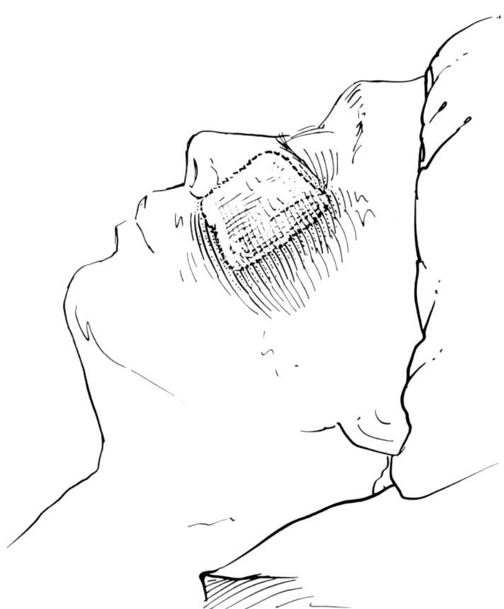

Figure 5-16

Iced-saline-soaked cotton gauzes placed over the cheeks as well as elevation of the head of the bed markedly reduce postoperative swelling (Figure 5-16).

TRANSANTRAL TECHNIQUE

Fractures of the malar bone may also be approached through a sublabial-transantral approach. This approach may be used separately or in conjunction with the percutaneous route in order to provide better mobilization and reduction of the malar fracture. There are no facial scars, and it is useful for comminuted fractures.

Lidocaine 1% with epinephrine 1:100,000 is infiltrated in the area of the planned incision (Figure 5-17). The patient's face is then prepared and draped.

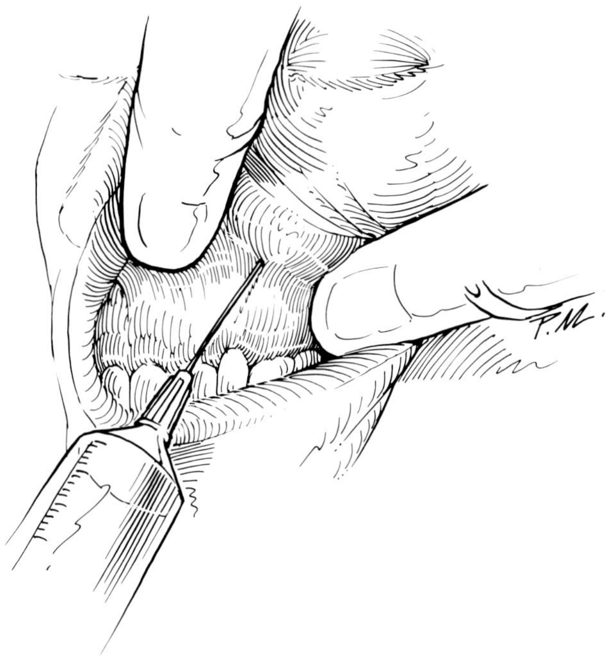

Figure 5-17

With the cheek retracted laterally, an incision is made in the gingivobuccal sulcus so that there will be enough mucosa on the alveolar side to allow for easy closure (Figure 5-18). The incision is carried through the mucosa, submucosa, and periosteum down to bone.

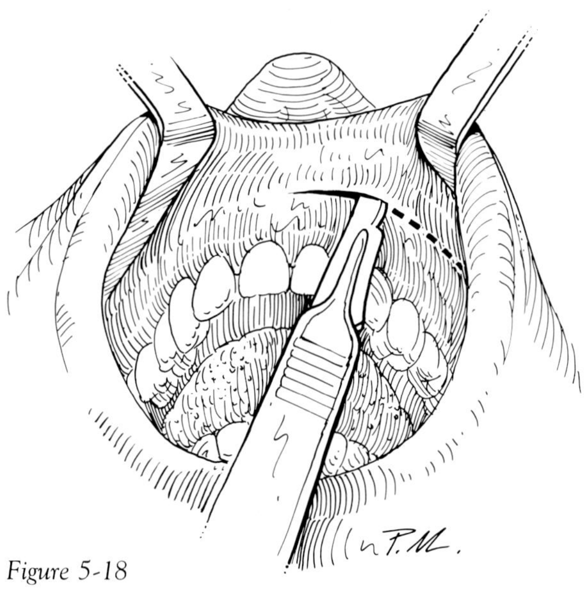

Figure 5-18

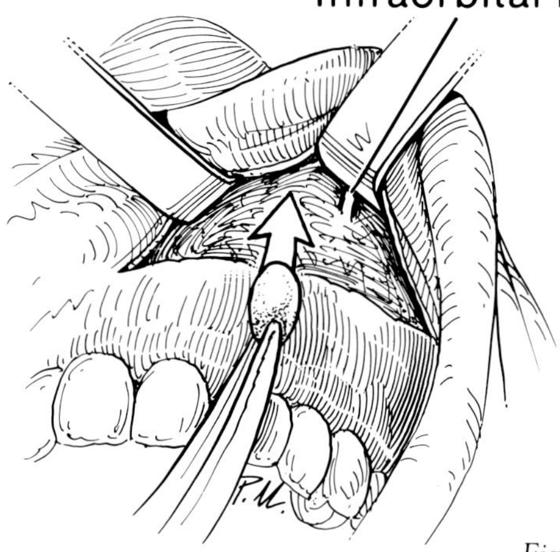

Figure 5-19

An elevator is used gently to elevate the periosteum (Figure 5-19). A Kittner dissector is used very effectively once the elevation has begun. The infraorbital nerve is identified, and the entire anterior wall of the maxillary sinus is exposed.

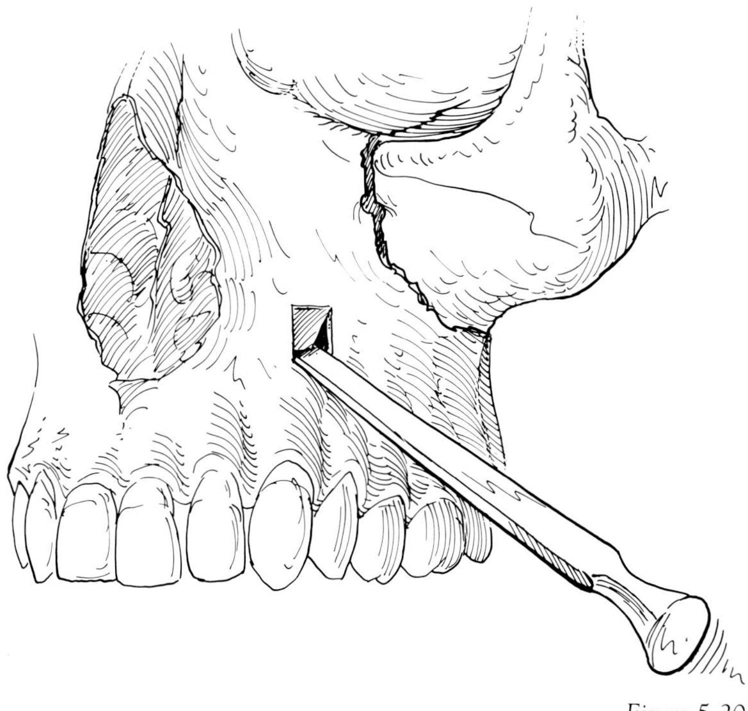

Figure 5-20

An osteotome is used to make a window measuring approximately 1 cm in the anterior wall of the maxillary sinus in the canine fossa (Figure 5-20).

The Kerrison rongeur is used to enlarge the opening to include the entire anterior wall of the maxillary sinus (Figure 5-21). Care is taken not to injure the infraorbital nerve.

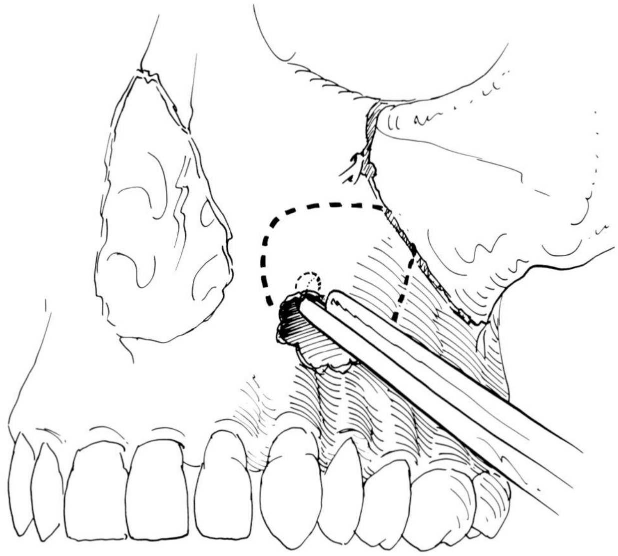

Figure 5-21

The orbital floor is carefully inspected. Any fragments of bone that are oriented vertically should be either removed or redirected so that they do not injure the globe during reduction (Figure 5-22).

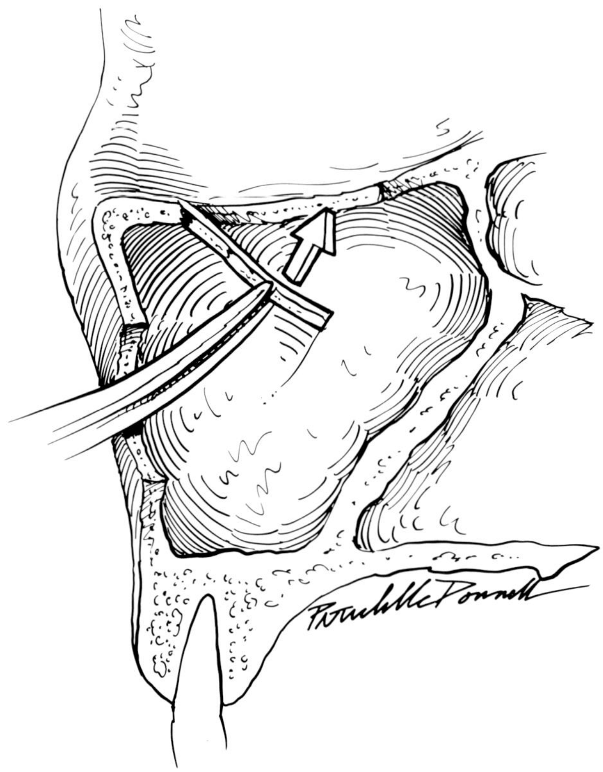

Figure 5-22

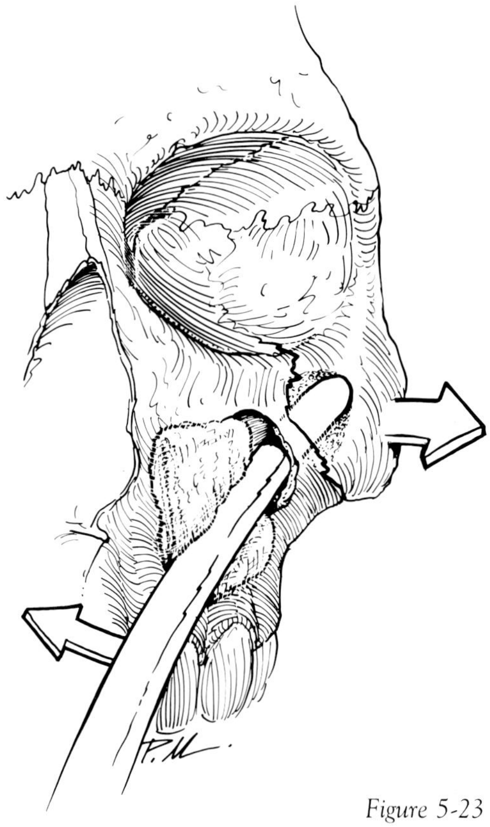

Figure 5-23

An elevator, urethral sound, or other instrument is placed in the lateral recess of the maxillary sinus to reduce the fracture to its normal position (Figure 5-23). Care must be taken to pad the area of the fulcrum so as not to injure other structures.

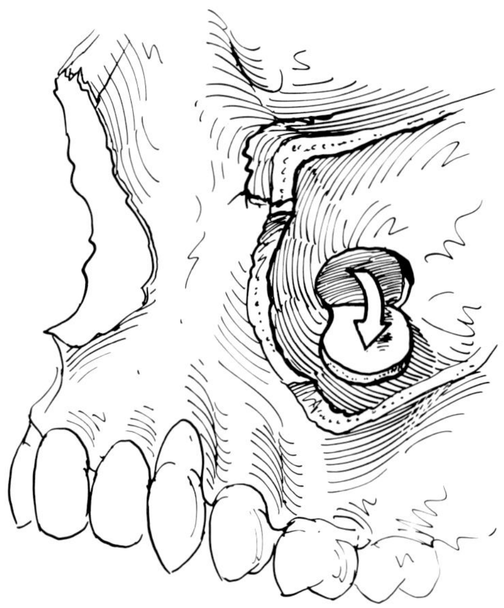

Figure 5-24

The osteotome is used to remove a 1-cm segment of bone in the area of the inferior meatus. An inferiorly based flap is created in the nasal mucosa (Figure 5-24).

A clamp is passed transnasally through the nasoantral window and the end of a segment of cotton gauze (Nu-gauze), which has been impregnated with antibiotic ointment, is grasped and pulled through the nose (Figure 5-25). The packing of the sinus begins in the lateral recess and progresses from lateral to medial, while the fracture reduction is carefully maintained. This allows for much easier and less painful removal of the packing.

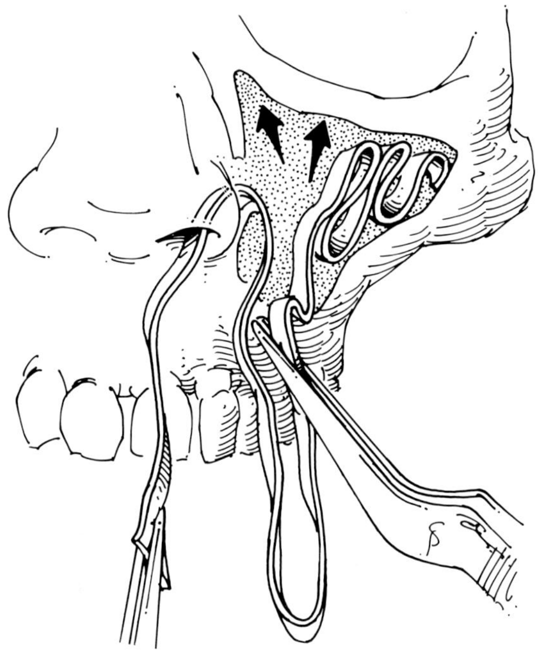

Figure 5-25

A forced duction test is performed to make sure that there has not been entrapment of the inferior rectus muscle during manipulation of the fracture (Figure 5-26).

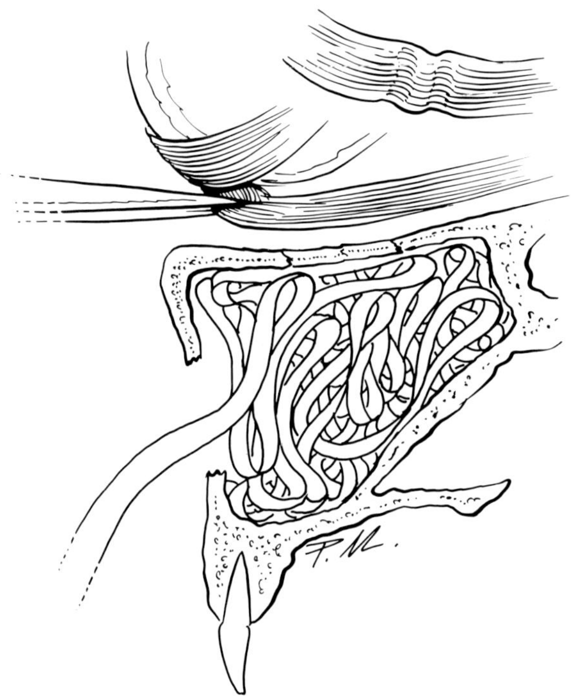

Figure 5-26

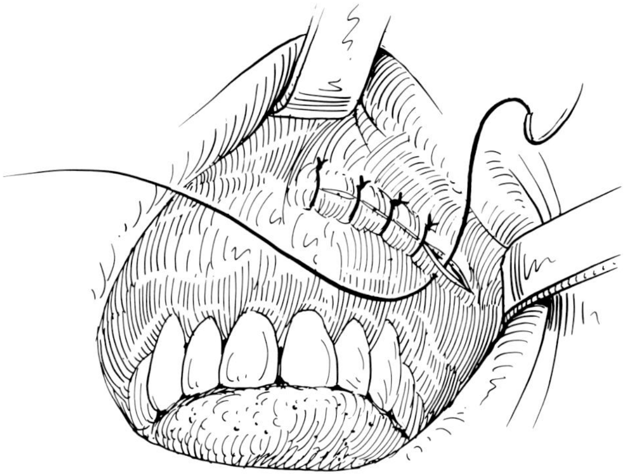

Figure 5-27

The intraoral incision is closed with absorbable sutures (Figure 5-27).

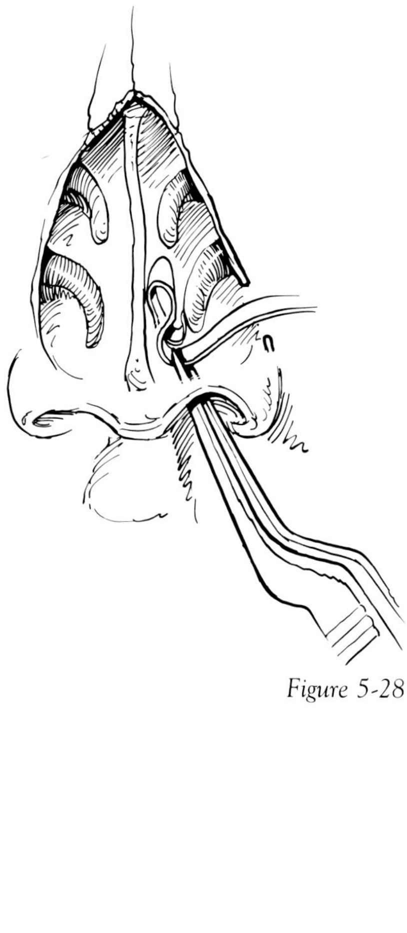

Figure 5-28

The portion of the Nu-gauze that had been pulled through the nasoantral window is lightly packed into the nose (Figure 5-28). The packing is removed 10 days postoperatively.

PIN TECHNIQUE

Another alternative treatment of a trimalar fracture utilizes a Steinmann pin for fixation. It is very useful for minimally displaced, noncomminuted fracture.

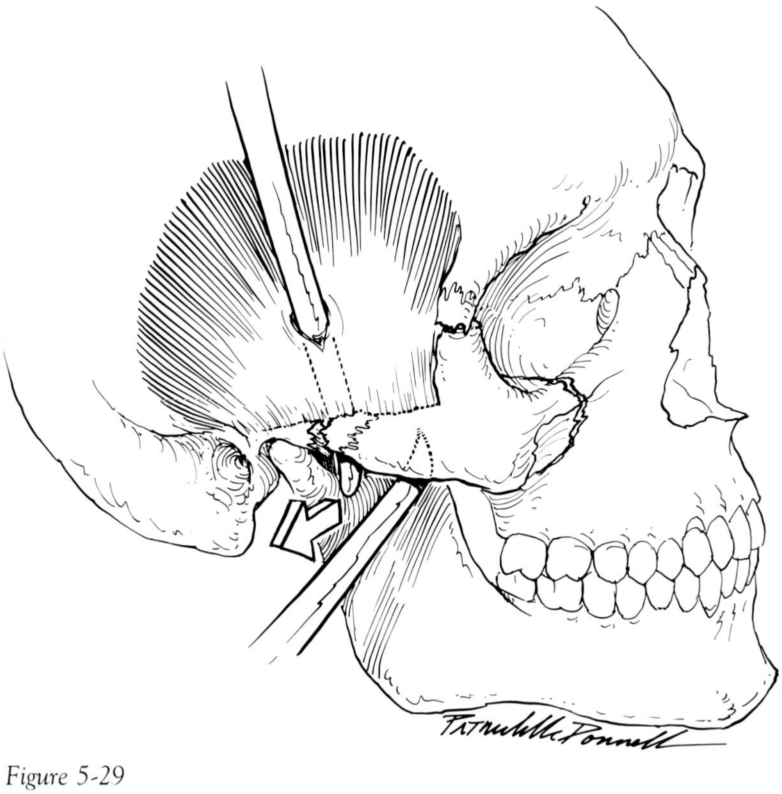

Figure 5-29

The fracture is reduced by Gillies' approach through the hairline or by a bone hook placed through a stab wound in the face (Figure 5-29).

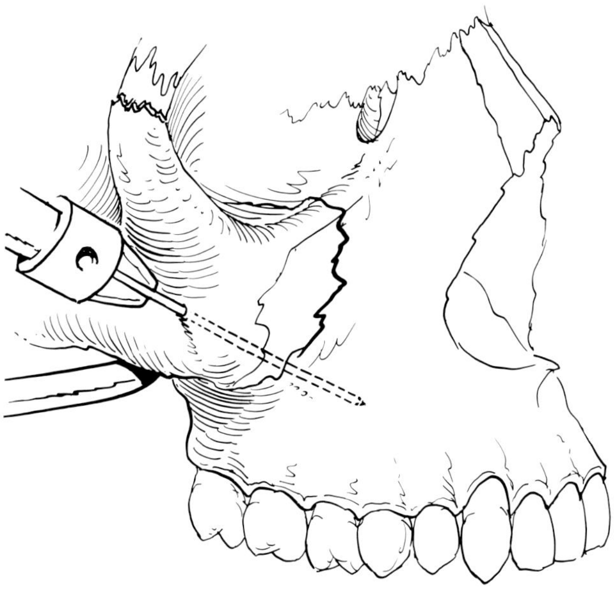

Figure 5-30

A small stab wound is made in the skin over the lateral aspect of the malar bone. While the reductions are carefully maintained with instruments and digital pressure, a 3/16-inch unthreaded Steinmann pin is drilled through the malar bone, passing through the antrum to the hard palate approximately 2 cm posterior to the anterior nasal spine (Figure 5-30).

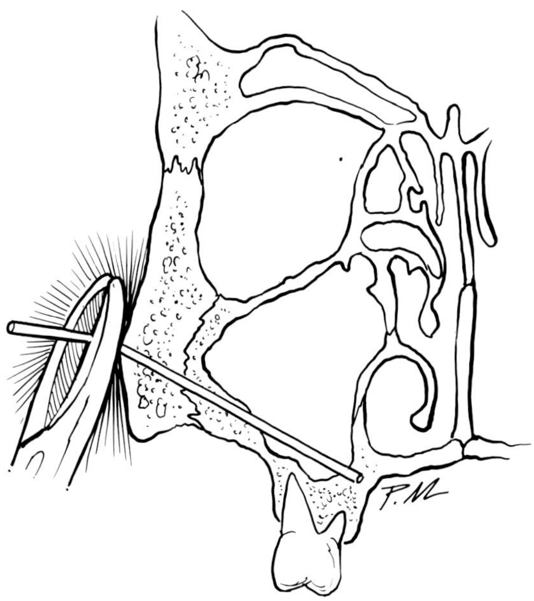

Figure 5-31

The metallic pin is transected flush with the skin (Figure 5-31), and the skin incisions are closed, if necessary.

Six weeks postoperatively a small skin incision is made over the pin, which is removed with a pair of pliers or other strong grasping instrument (Figure 5-32).

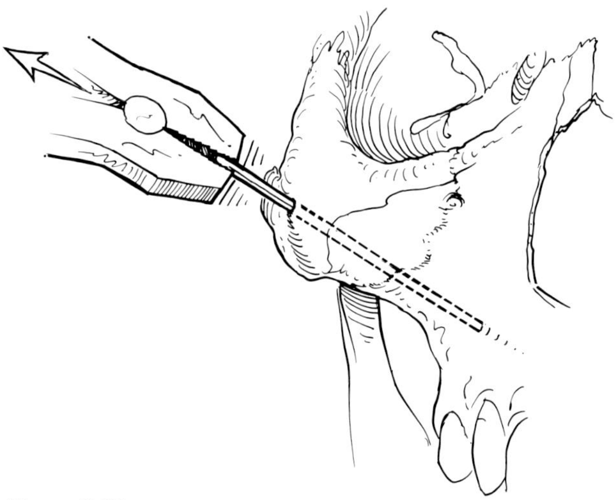

Figure 5-32

ZYGOMATIC ARCH FRACTURES

GILLIES' TECHNIQUE

Elevation of isolated zygomatic arch fractures can be accomplished through Gillies' approach. An incision is made in the sideburn area and carried through the temporalis fascia (Figure 5-33). Since the temporalis fascia attaches to the zygomatic arch, the elevator must be deep to the fascia in order to pass under the zygomatic arch. An incision in the lateral eyebrow can also be used similarly to approach the zygoma and the arch.

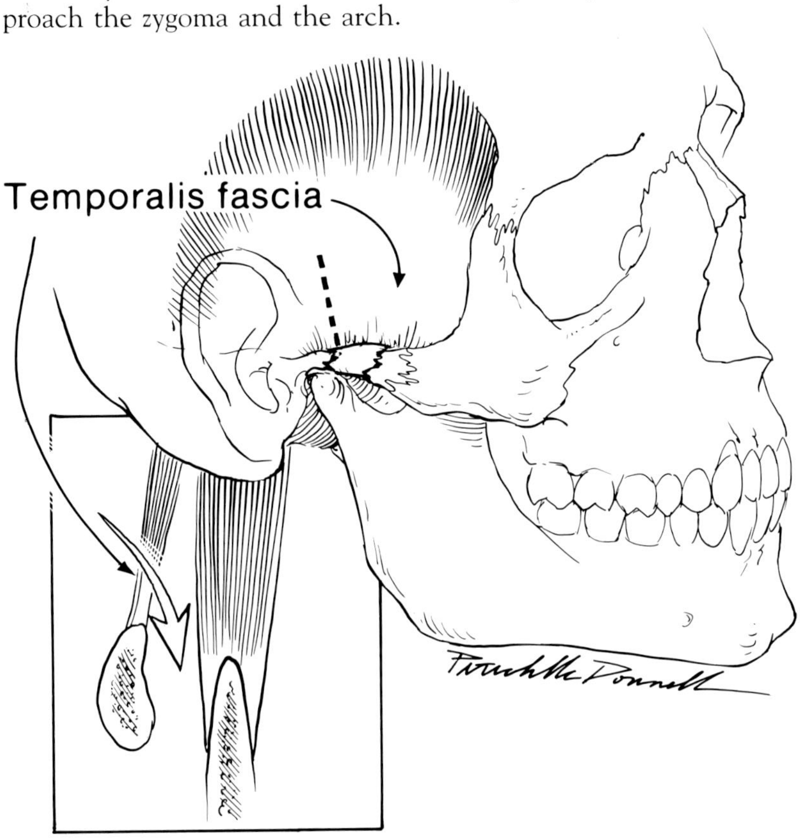

Figure 5-33

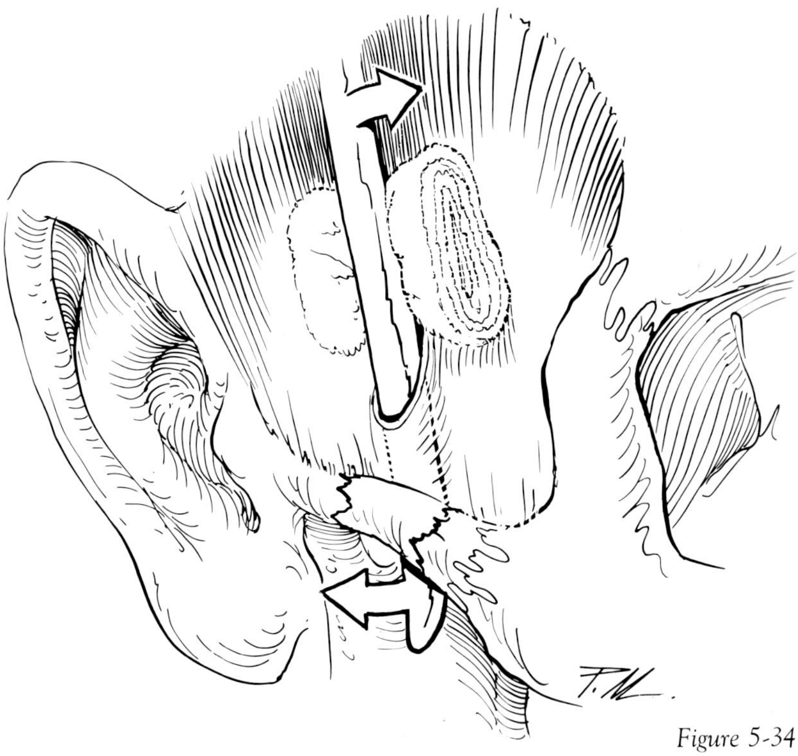

Figure 5-34

A strong instrument such as a urethral sound is passed under the zygomatic arch and, with a rolled sponge placed as padding in the area of the fulcrum, the zygomatic arch is elevated (Figure 5-34).

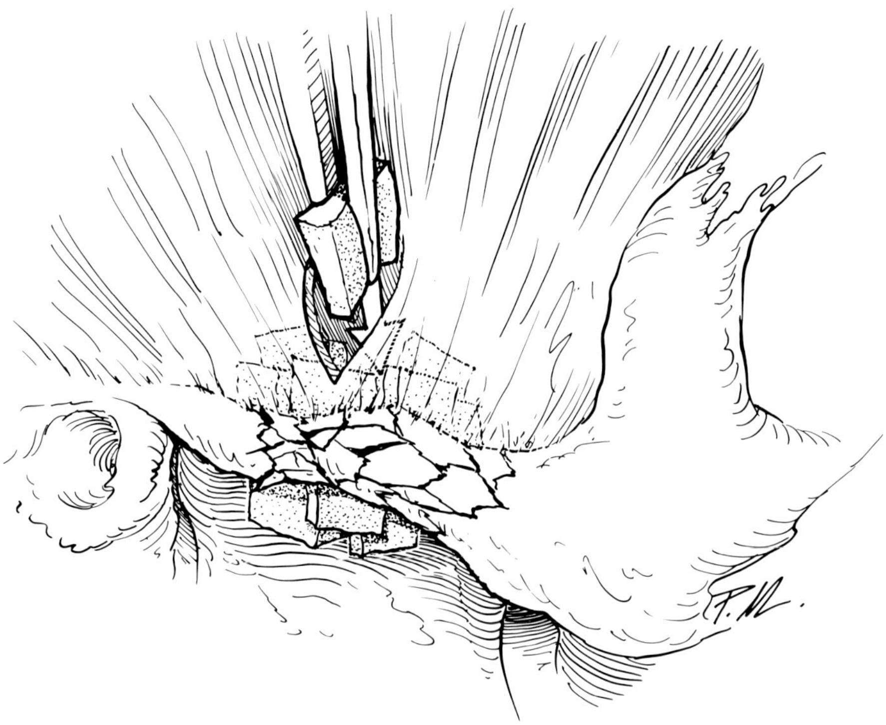

Figure 5-35

Packing of the arch in its normal position is usually not necessary; however, should the arch continue to collapse following reduction, Gelfoam can be packed into the area in order to maintain the arch in its normal position (Figure 5-35).

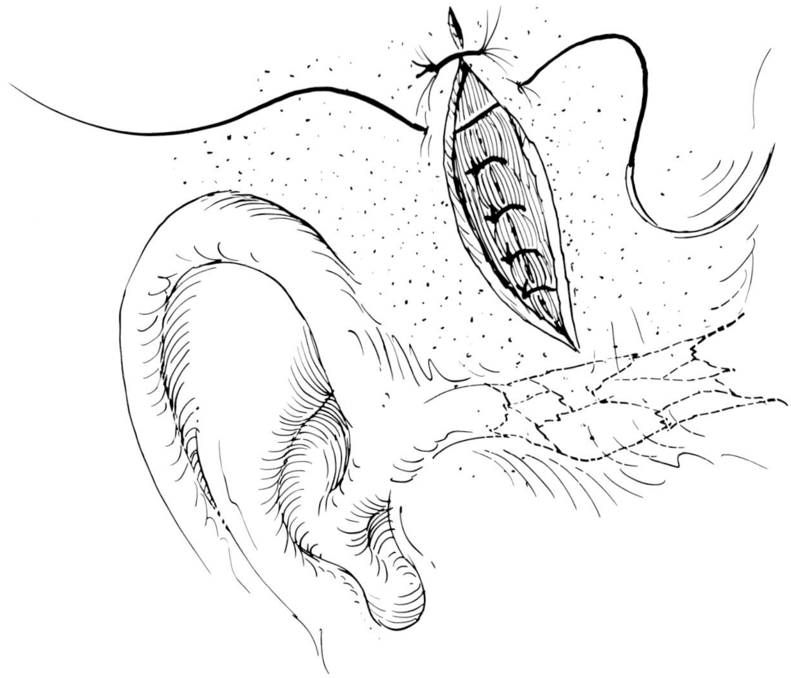

Figure 5-36

The fascia is closed with absorbable sutures and the skin is closed with nonabsorbable sutures (Figure 5-36).

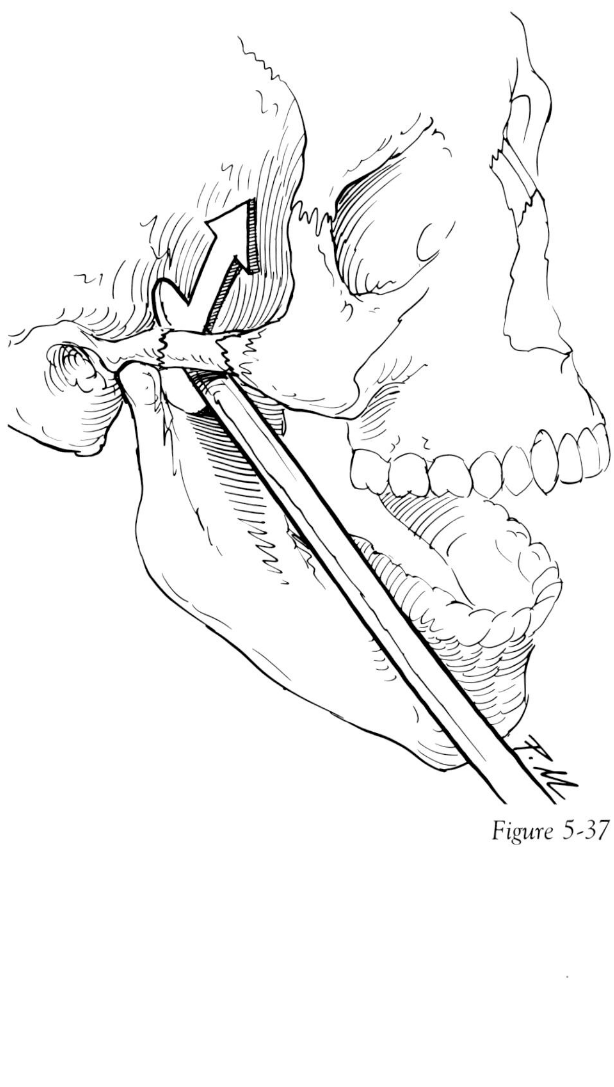

Figure 5-37

ALTERNATIVE TECHNIQUES AND SPECIAL CASES

Another approach to isolated zygomatic arch fractures is to make an incision in the superior gingivobuccal sulcus and pass an elevator deep to the arch (Figure 5-37).

Open reduction and internal fixation of an isolated zygomatic arch fracture is rarely indicated. When necessary, however, it can be accomplished through a horizontal incision over the zygomatic arch with direct wiring of the fragments (Figure 5-38). Care must be taken to avoid injury to the frontal branch of the facial nerve, which crosses the area of the incision.

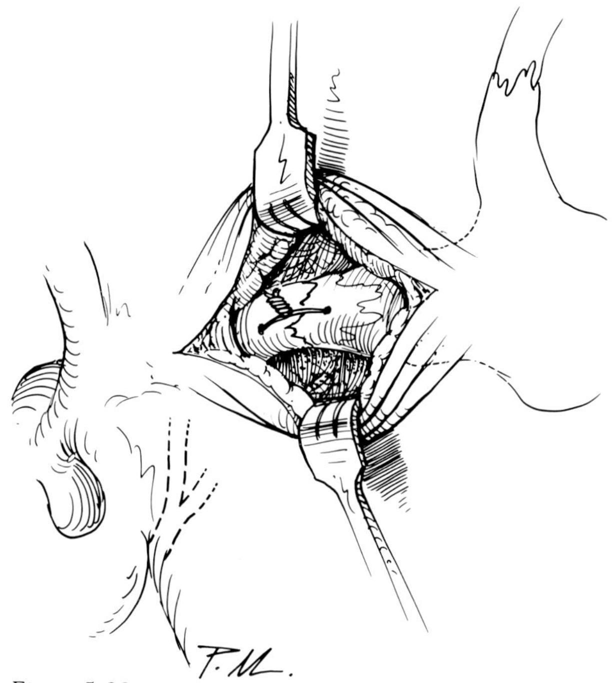

Figure 5-38

REFERENCES

1. Gillies, H. D., Kilner, T. P., and Stone, D.: Fractures of the Malarzygomatic Compound; With Description of a New X-Ray Position. *Br. J. Surg.*, 14:651–656, 1927.
2. Lothrop, H. A.: Fractures of the Superior Maxillary Bone Caused by Direct Blows over the Malar Bone. *Boston Med. Surg. J.*, 154:8–14, 1906.
3. Matsunaga, R. S., Simpson, W., and Toffel, P. H.: Simplified Protocol for Treatment of Malar Fractures. *Arch. Otolaryngol.*, 103:535–538, 1977.

6
Fractures of the Orbital Floor

PERCUTANEOUS TECHNIQUE

Isolated fractures of the orbital floor can be explored externally through an infraciliary incision or an incision through an existing skin crease (Figure 6-1).

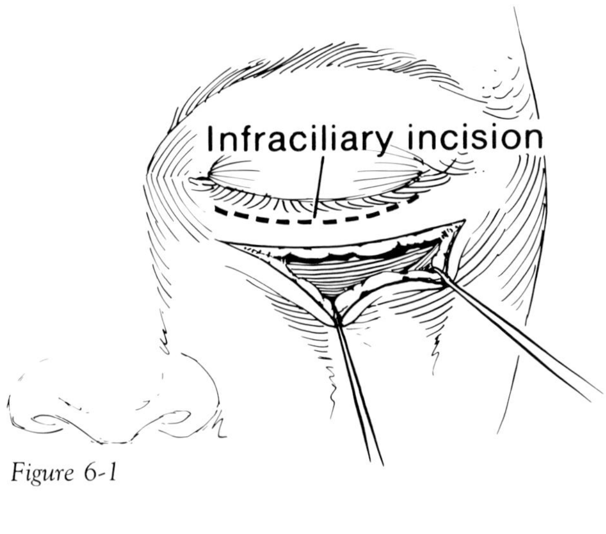

Figure 6-1

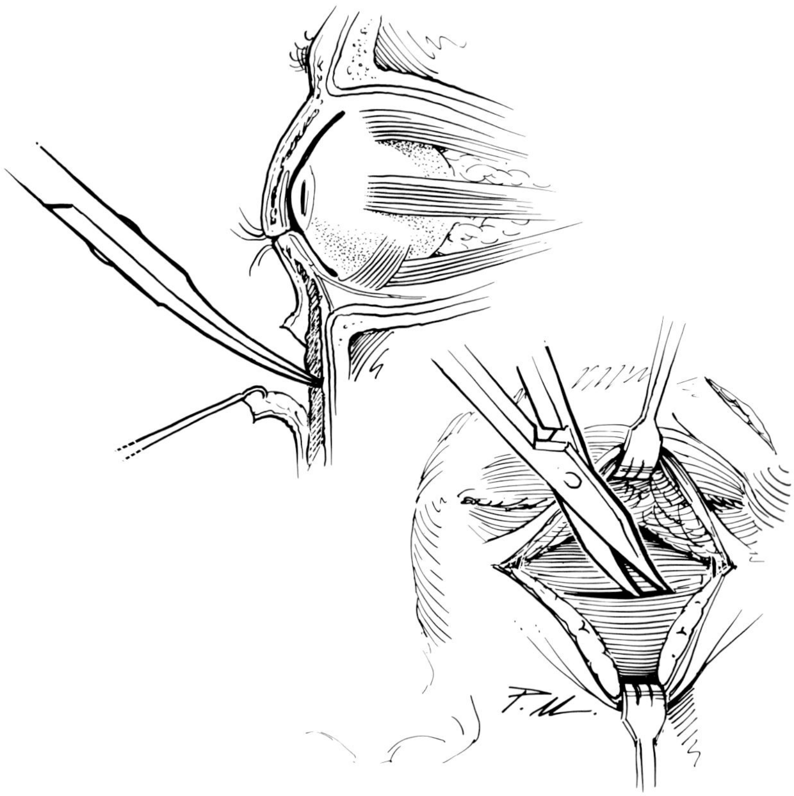

Figure 6-2

A skin flap is elevated inferiorly, and the orbicularis oculi muscle is divided bluntly to expose the infraorbital rim (Figure 6-2). The incidence of ectropion is reduced by placing the muscle incision at a different level than the skin incision.

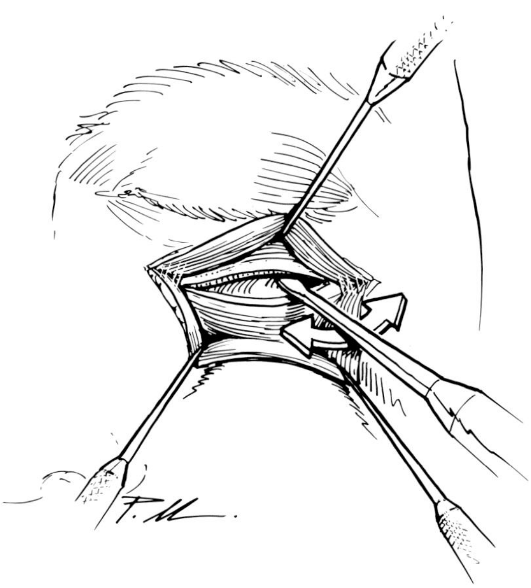

An incision is made in the periosteum along the infraorbital rim (Figure 6-3).

Figure 6-3

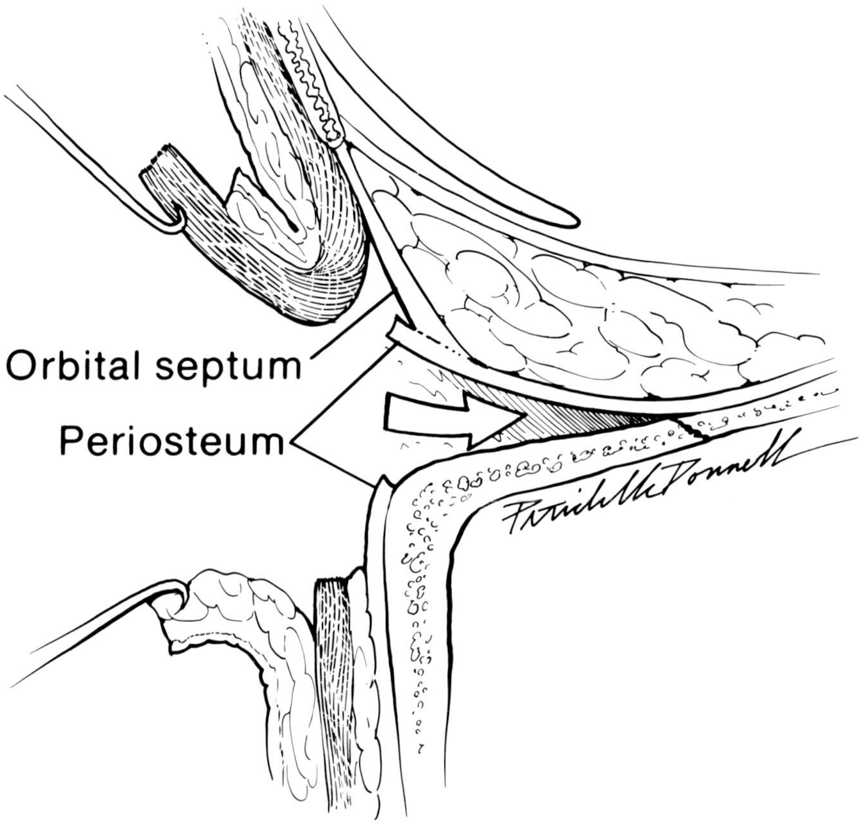

Figure 6-4

Periostial elevators are used to elevate the periosteum off the orbital floor (Figure 6-4). Extreme care is taken not to injure the periosteum, as this would allow orbital fat to herniate into the area, making the dissection more difficult.

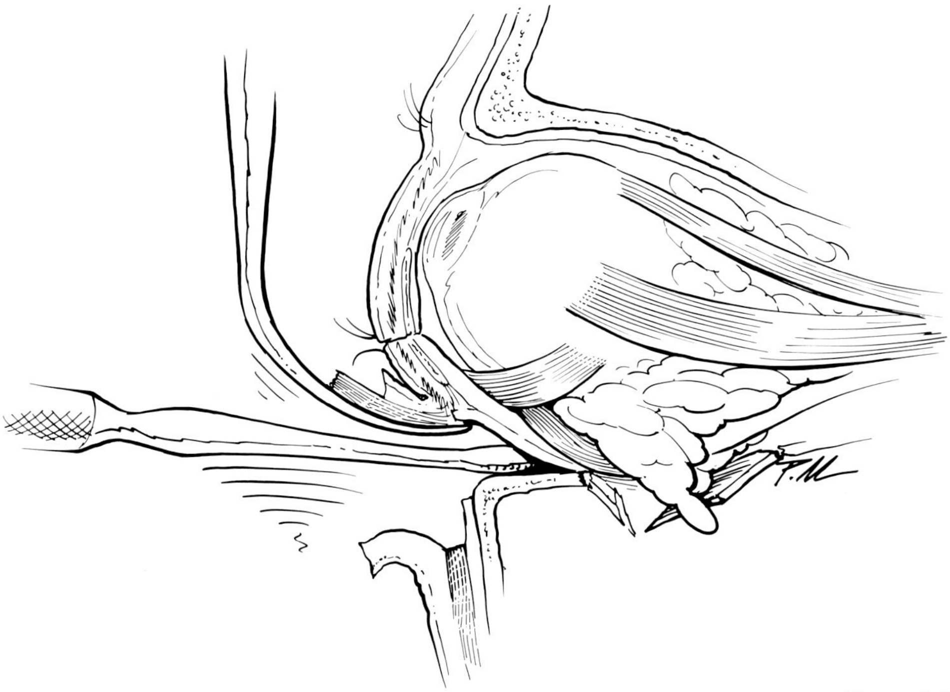

Figure 6-5

Orbital retractors are used carefully to retract the orbit, and the orbital floor is examined (Figure 6-5). Any entrapped orbital contents, such as fat or inferior rectus muscle, are carefully teased from the fracture line and returned to their normal positions.

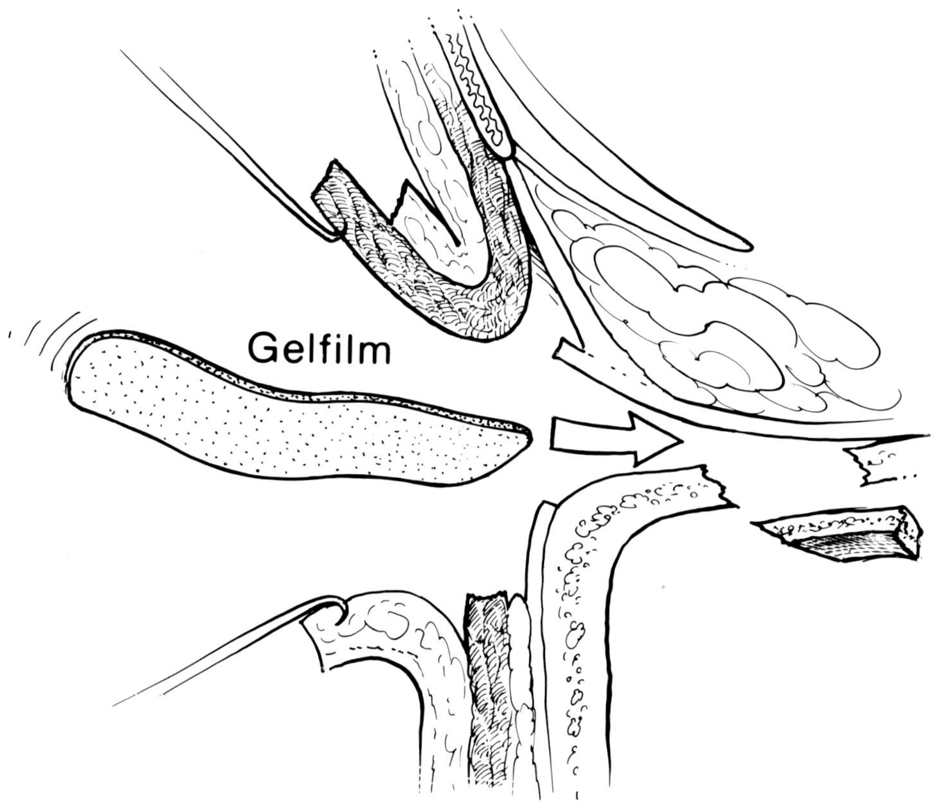

Figure 6-6

If the fracture is small, then a piece of Gelfilm can be used to reconstruct the orbital floor (Figure 6-6).

Larger defects should be repaired with Teflon or Silastic sheeting with a notch cut anteriorly to help hold the implant in place (Figure 6-7). Care is taken so that the implant does not impinge on the optic nerve posteriorly.

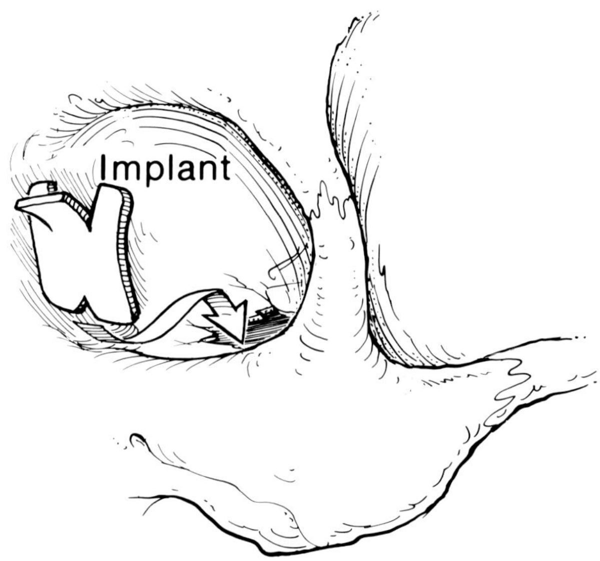

Figure 6-7

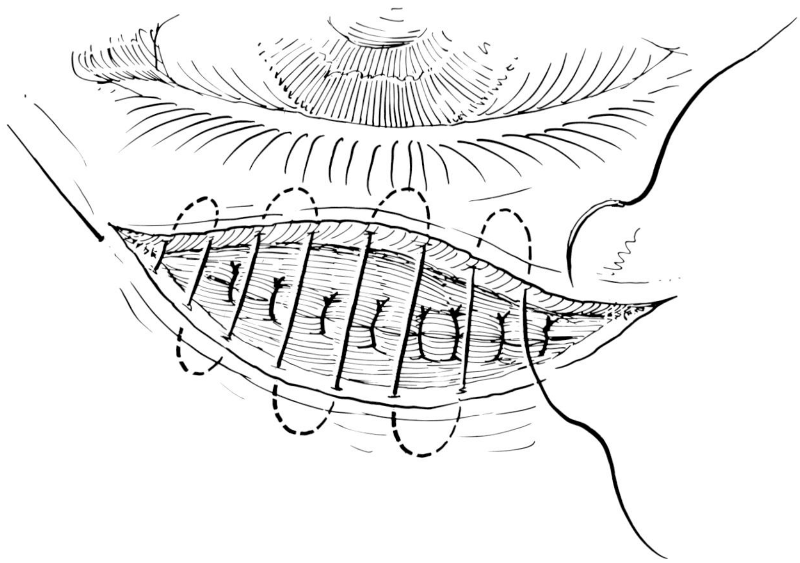

Figure 6-8

The periosteum is closed with interrupted sutures, and the skin is closed with a subcuticular suture (Figure 6-8).

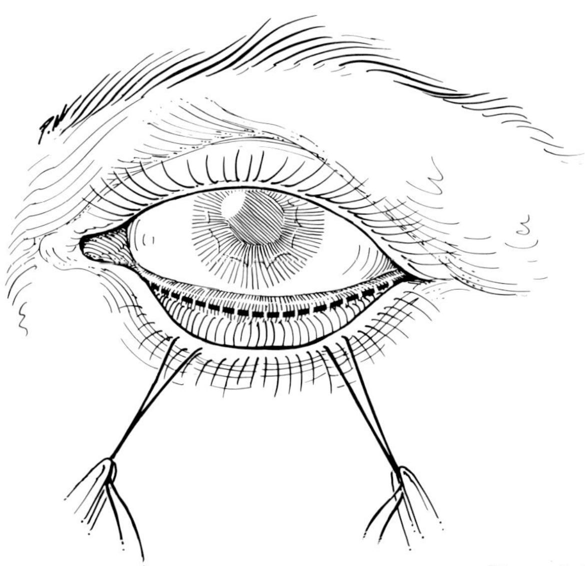

Figure 6-9

CONJUNCTIVAL TECHNIQUE

Another approach to orbital floor fractures is the conjunctival approach. Although the exposure is somewhat limited, this approach does avoid the minimal facial scar associated with a cutaneous approach.

The lower eyelid is retracted inferiorly, and a conjunctival incision is made at the lower border of the tarsal plate (Figure 6-9).

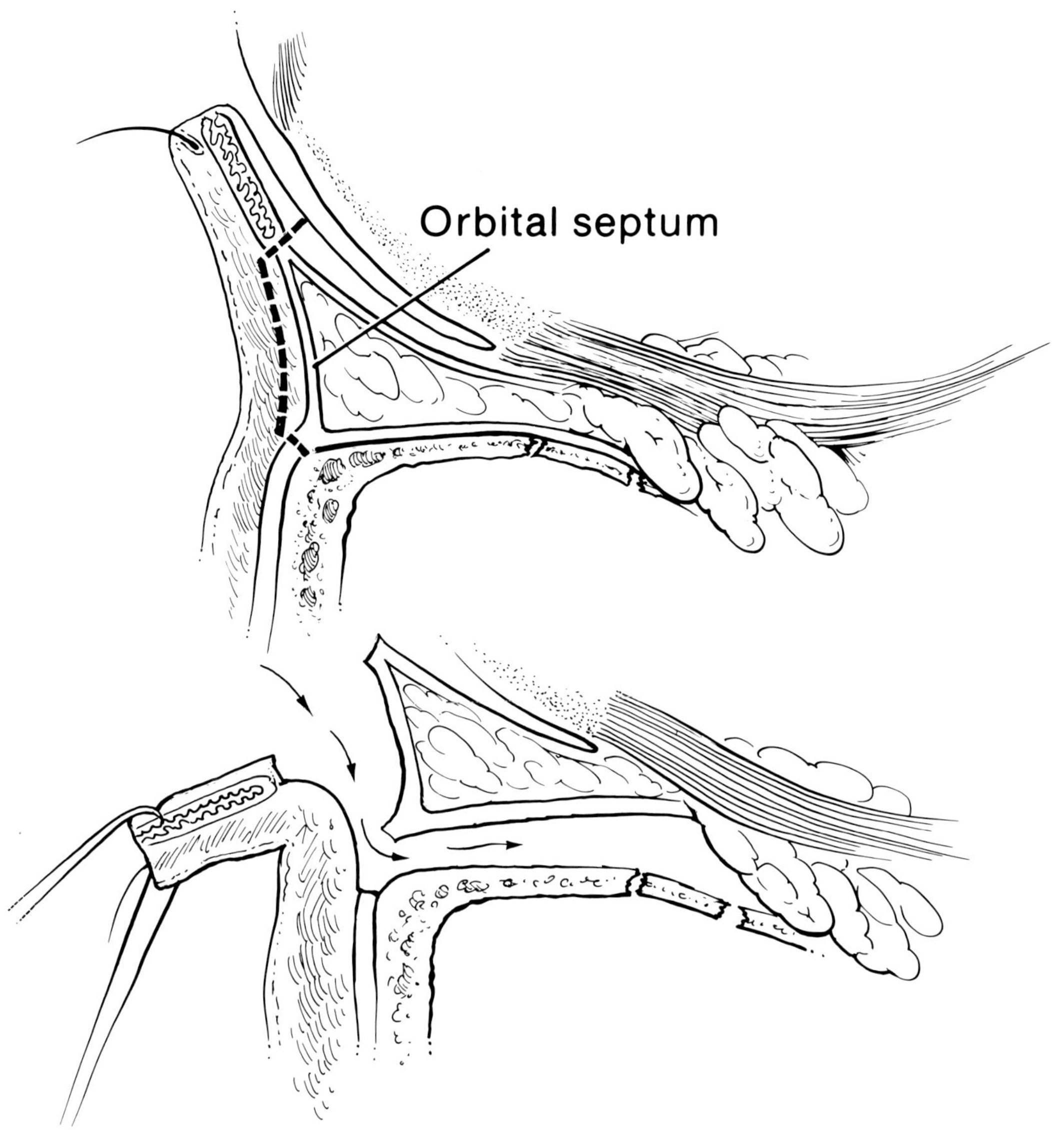

Figure 6-10

In the preseptal approach the orbital septum is separated from the lower border of the tarsal plate, and dissection is carried down to the orbital floor anterior to the orbital septum (Figure 6-10).

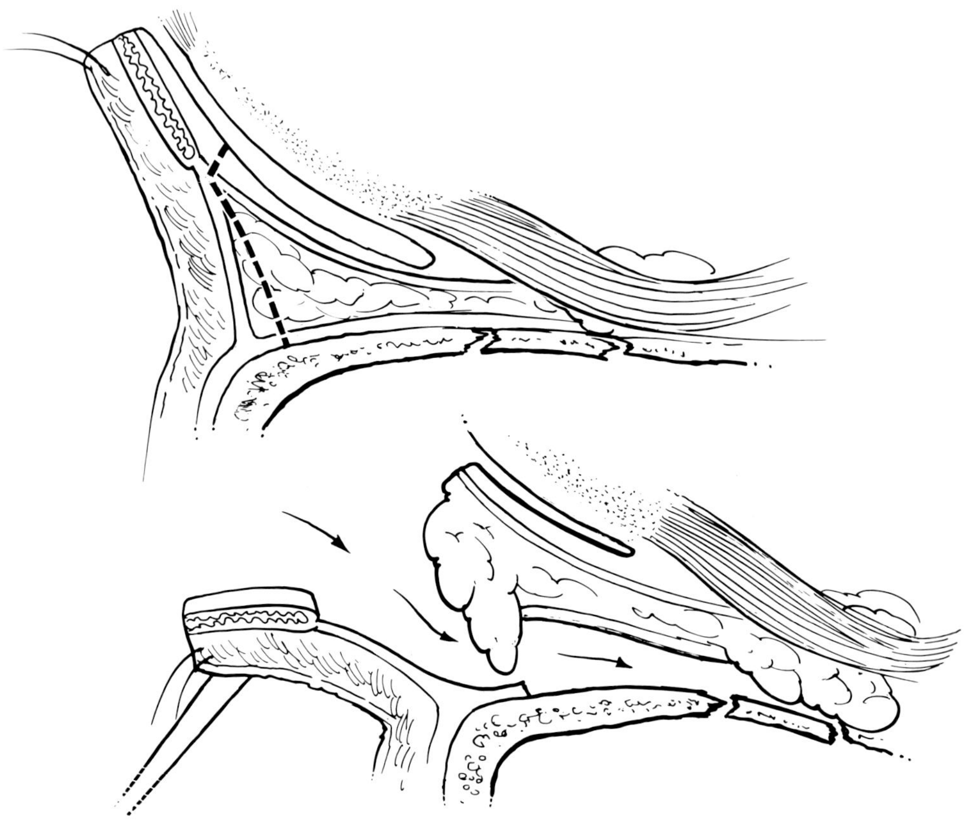

Figure 6-11

In the retroseptal approach the dissection is carried just posterior to the orbital septum directly to the orbital floor (Figure 6-11). The disadvantage of the retroseptal approach is that the orbital fat is exposed and is difficult to retract out of the operative field. The orbital floor fracture is then repaired in the same fashion as described for the percutaneous technique.

REFERENCES

1. Converse, J. M., Firmin, F., Wood-Smith, D., *et al.*: The Conjunctival Approach in Orbital Fractures. *Plast. Reconstr. Surg.*, 52:656–657, 1973.
2. Converse, J. M. and Smith, B.: Blowout Fractures of the Orbital Floor. *Trans. Am. Acad. Ophthalmol. Otolaryngol.*, 64:676–688, 1960.

7
Fractures of the Maxilla and Naso-orbital Region

LEFORT FRACTURES

Although LeFort fractures can be quite severe, proper treatment usually provides very satisfactory results. The basic concept in repairing LeFort fractures is to provide suspension from a stable point superiorly and support from an intact mandible inferiorly. Intermaxillary fixation not only provides immobilization but also serves as a guide for proper positioning of the mobile midface. It is crucial to assess the status of the zygomatic arches, as this determines how the fracture is suspended superiorly.

In the LeFort I and II fractures the zygomatic arch is intact and consequently can be used for stabilization (Figure 7-1). Since the zygomatic arch is involved in the LeFort III fracture, suspension must be accomplished from a more superior stable bone.

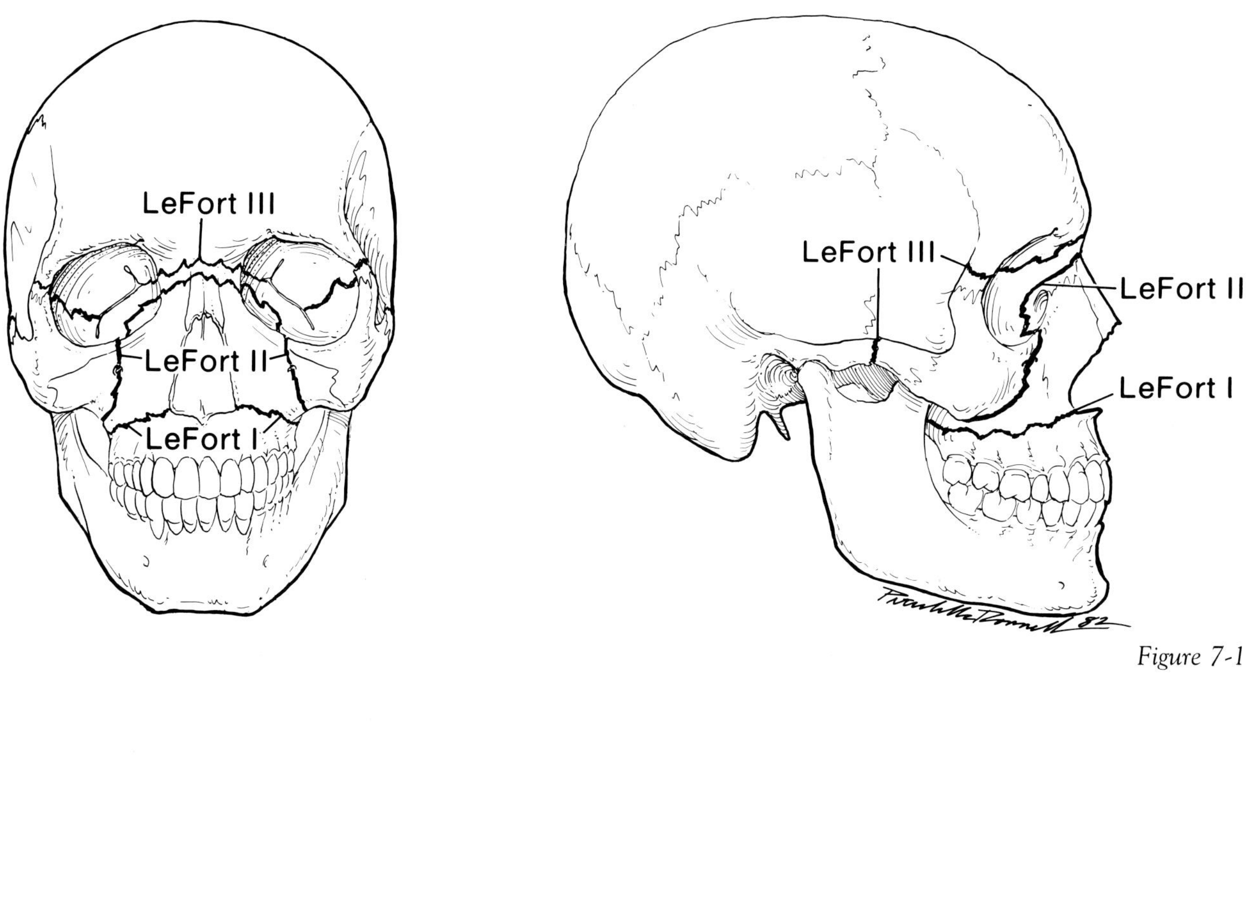

Figure 7-1

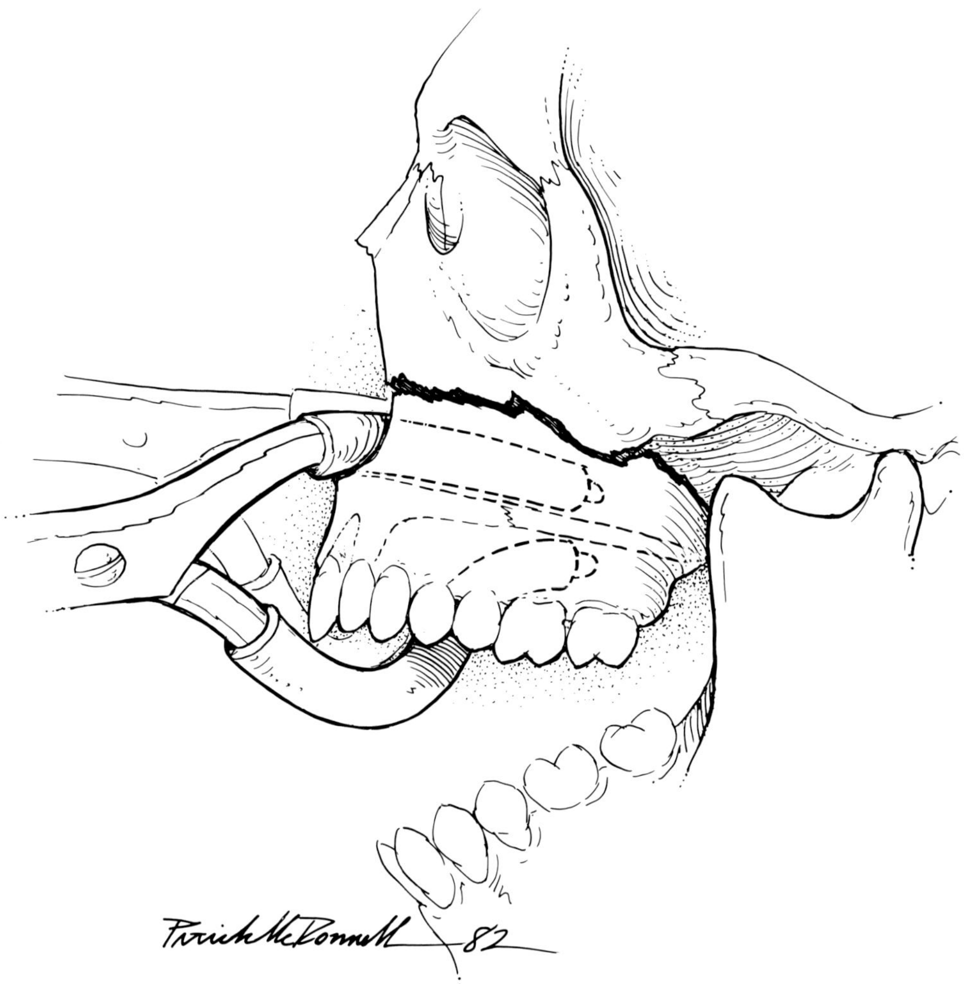

Figure 7-2

If the maxilla is impacted, Rowe's disimpaction forceps are used to achieve reduction (Figure 7-2).

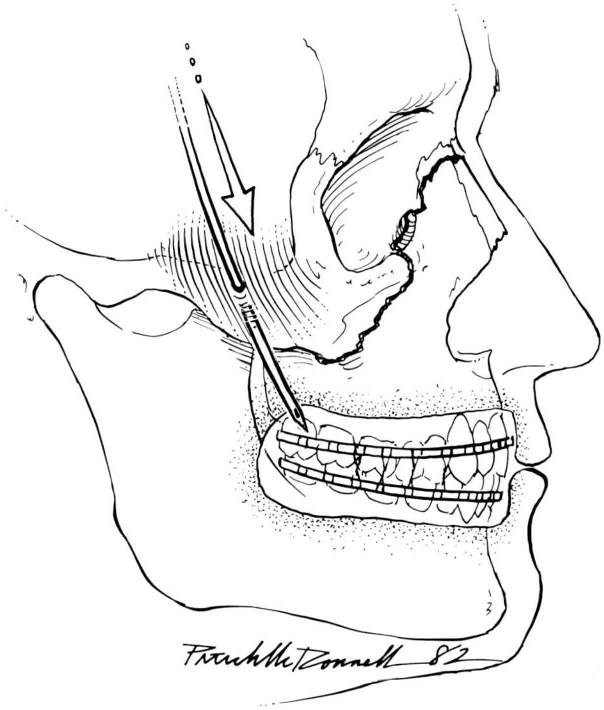

Figure 7-3

The first step in repairing a LeFort fracture is to obtain intermaxillary fixation as described in Chapter 2. Suspension from the zygomatic arch is achieved by passing an awl through the skin of the cheek lateral to the zygomatic arch and perforating the oral mucosa near the posterior aspect of the upper arch bar (Figure 7-3).

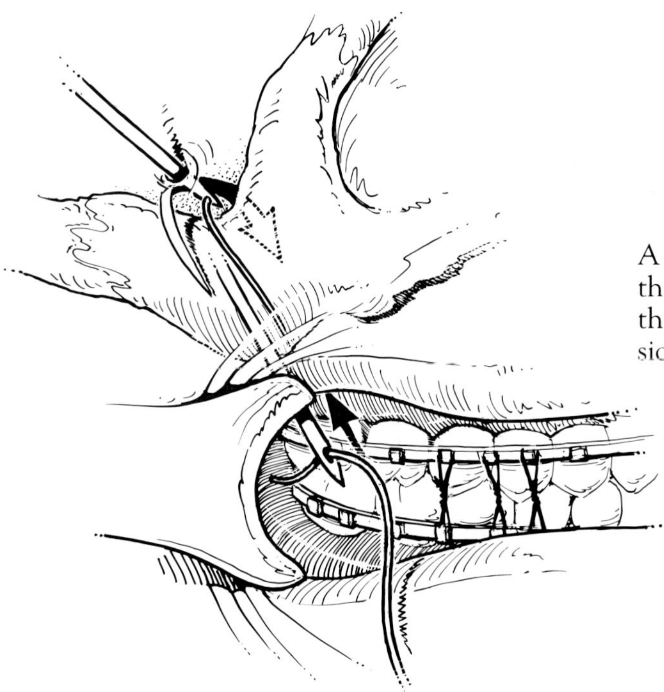

Figure 7-4

A wire is passed through the eye of the awl, and the awl is carefully withdrawn to a point just above the zygomatic arch without exiting the skin incision (Figure 7-4).

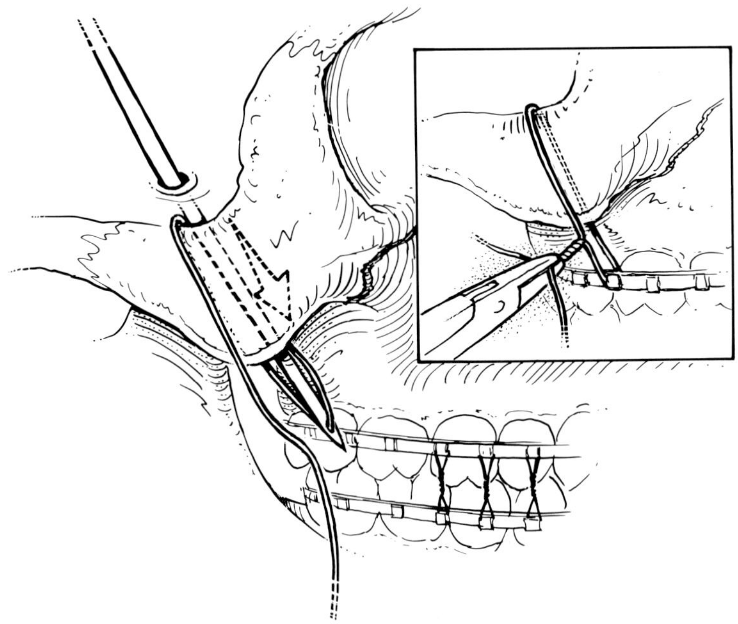

Figure 7-5

The awl then passes medial to the zygomatic arch and enters the oral cavity in the same area of the previous mucosal perforation (Figure 7-5). The wire is freed from the awl, which is withdrawn. The wire is then secured to the upper arch bar.

Some surgeons prefer to twist the circum-zygomatic wire so that it becomes a loop unattached to the upper arch bar. A second wire is then passed around the arch bar and twisted until the proper tension is achieved (Figure 7-6). With this technique only the small loop around the arch bar will break if too much tension is applied and it is very easily replaced.

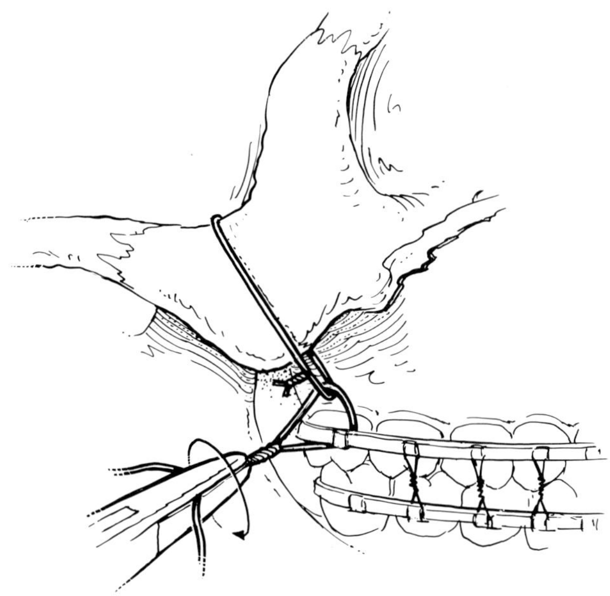

Figure 7-6

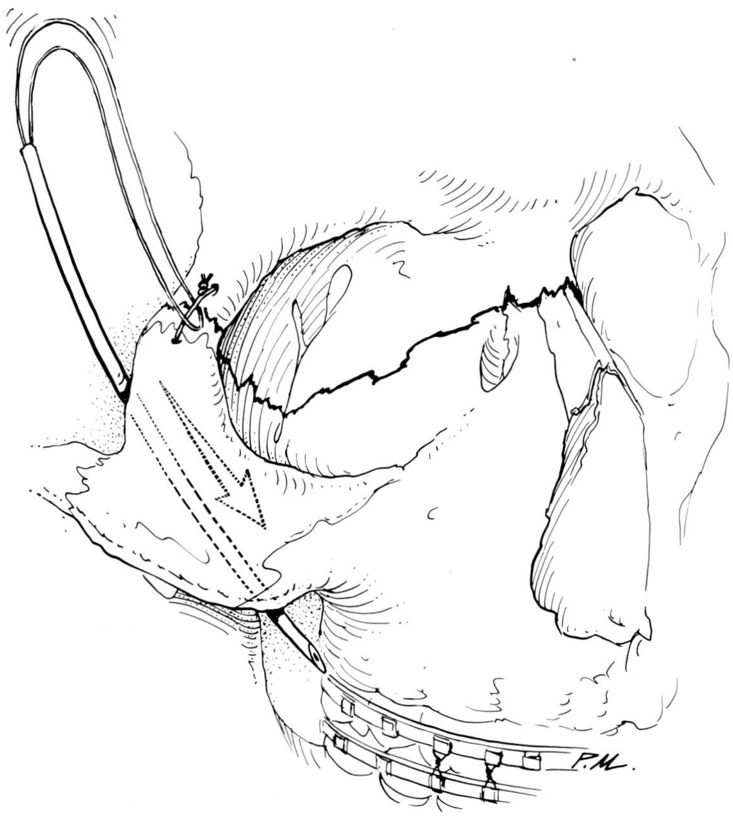

Figure 7-7

In the patient with a LeFort III fracture, suspension is achieved by reducing the zygomaticofrontal fracture and then passing the drop wire through the wire in the zygomatic process of the frontal bone (Figure 7-7). The wires are passed through a Dingman needle, which is passed through the soft tissue deep to the zygomatic arch. This drop wire is attached to the upper arch bar in a fashion identical to that used for the LeFort I and II fractures.

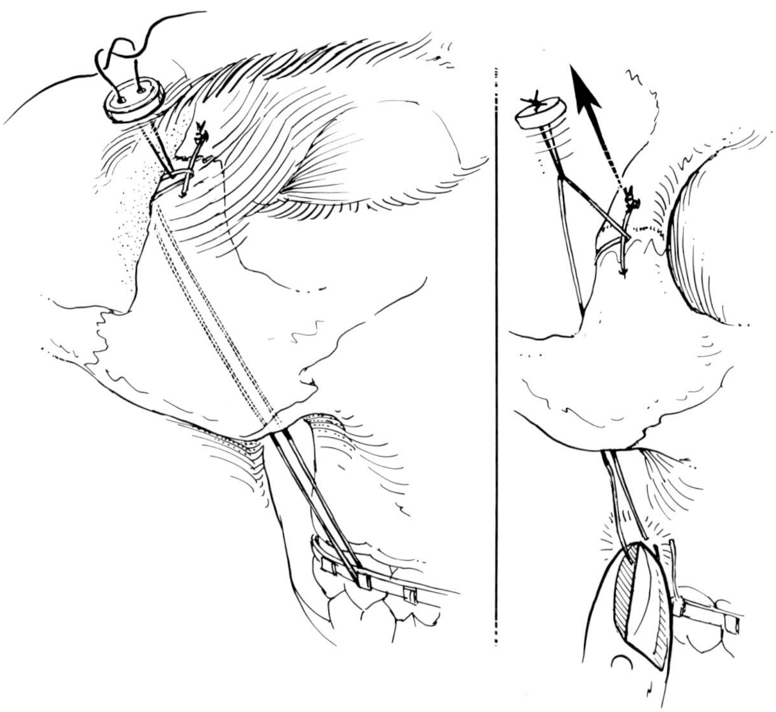

Figure 7-8

A pull-out wire is looped around the drop wire and affixed to a plastic button in the eyebrow (Figure 7-8). When the drop wire is to be removed, the intraoral loop is cut, and traction on the pull-out wire provides easy removal of the drop wire.

ALTERNATIVE TECHNIQUES

Some surgeons prefer to perform an open reduction and internal fixation of LeFort I fractures. An incision is made in the superior gingivobuccal sulcus and carried through the periosteum. The periosteum is elevated until the fracture is exposed. The fracture is reduced and the fragments wired together with stainless steel wire (Figure 7-9).

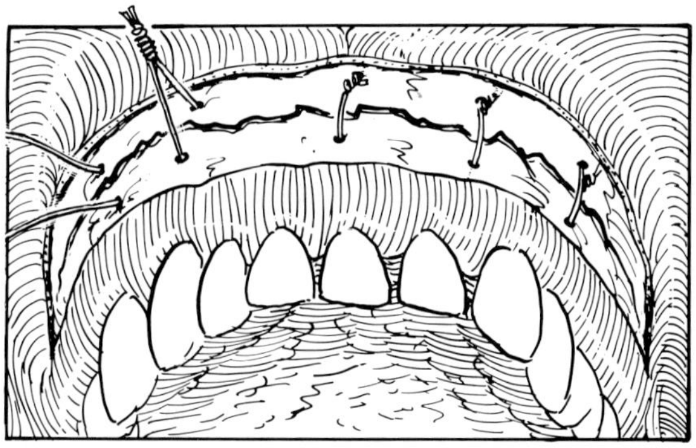

Figure 7-9

MEDIAL CANTHAL LIGAMENT INJURIES

Separation of the medial canthal ligament from its attachment to the medial orbital rim causes significant deformity. It should be repaired at the same time that the facial fracture is reduced, as late repair does not produce completely satisfactory results.

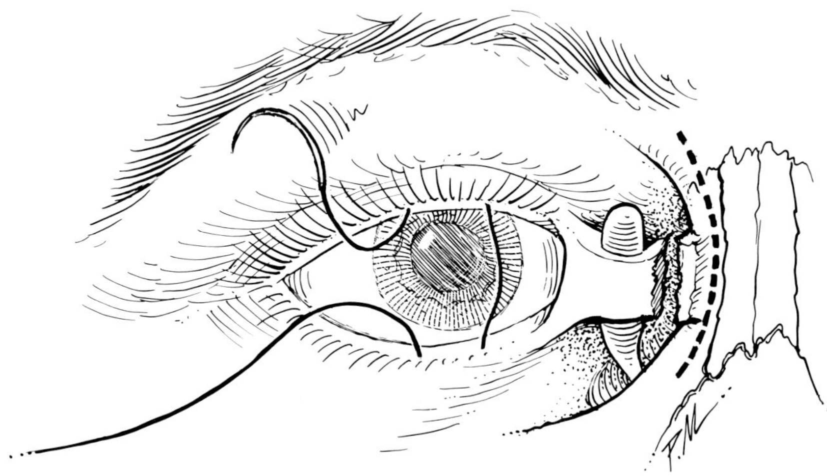

Figure 7-10

A tarsorrhaphy suture is placed to protect the globe (Figure 7-10). An incision is made one-half the distance between the dorsum of the nose and the medial canthus.

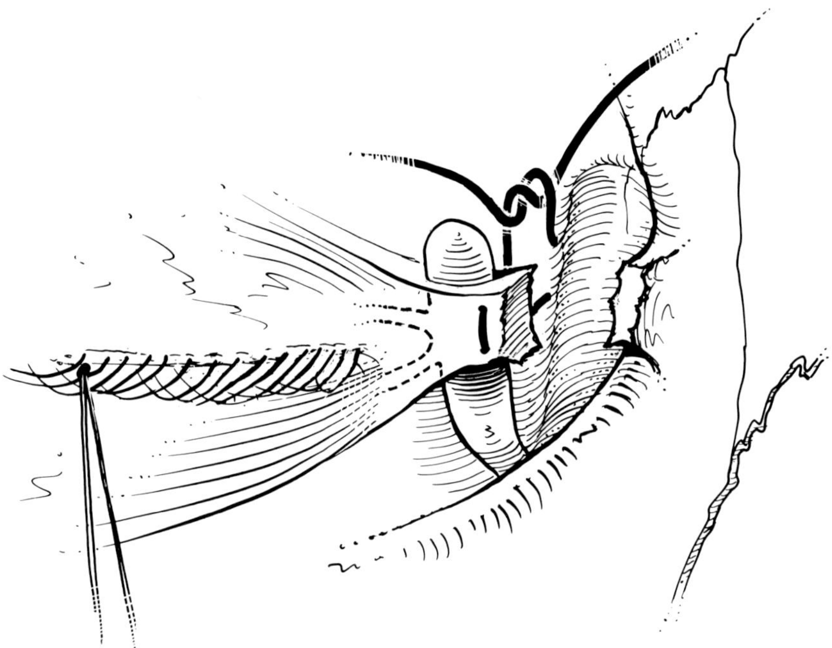

Figure 7-11

The medial canthal ligament is identified as its anterior and posterior bands pass around the lacrimal sac (Figure 7-11). A wire is passed through the ligament and then attached to the posterior lacrimal crest.

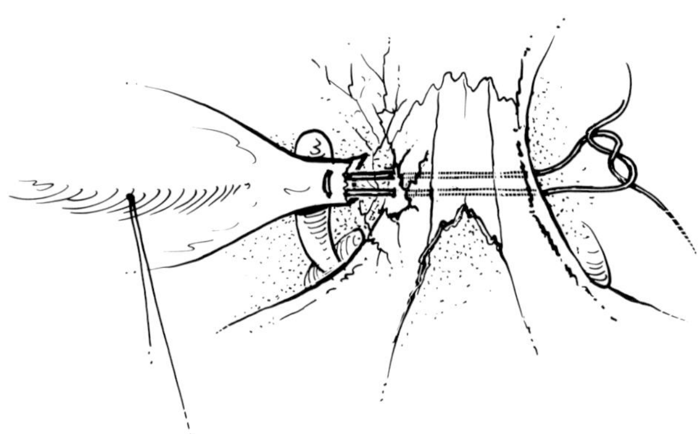

Figure 7-12

SPECIAL CASES

If the fracture of the medial orbital wall is so severe that stabilization of the ligament is not possible, then a wire can be passed through the nose and stabilized to the opposite lacrimal crest (Figure 7-12).

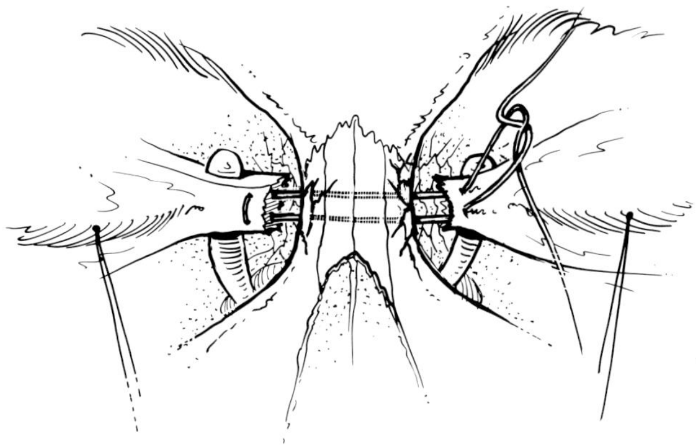

Figure 7-13

In bilateral medial canthal ligament injuries, the wire can be passed through both medial canthal ligaments in such a fashion that attachment to stable bone is not necessary (Figure 7-13).

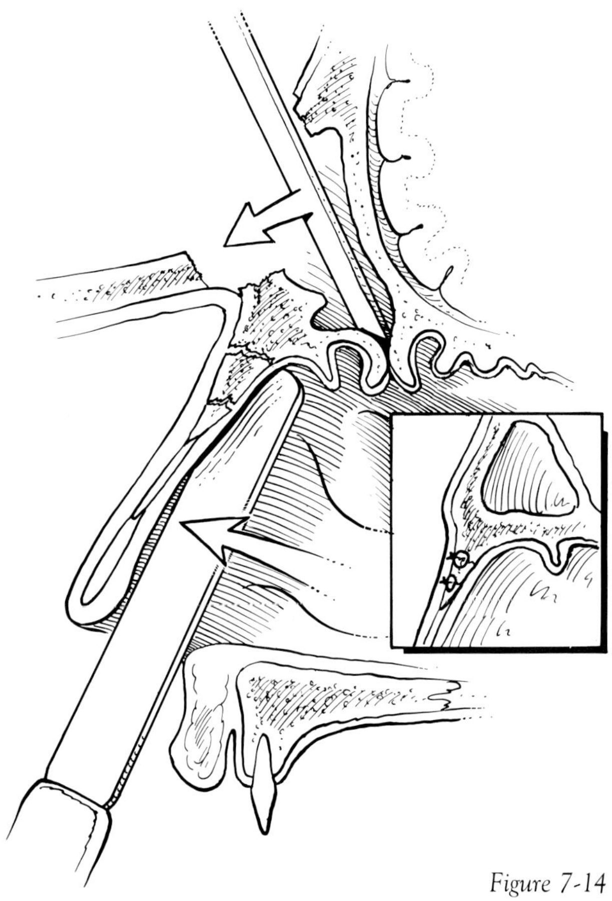

Figure 7-14

NASOFRONTOETHMOID FRACTURES

Nasofrontoethmoid fractures are unusual fractures in which the nasoethmoid complex is displaced posteriorly with a concomitant fracture of the frontal sinus. In addition to reduction of the nasoethmoid complex for cosmetic reasons, obliteration of the frontal sinus should be carried out since there is almost invariably a fracture involving at least the floor of the frontal sinus.

The frontal sinus is exposed through a coronal incision, and an osteoplastic flap is elevated (see Chapter 4). Elevators are placed in the nose as well as the nasofrontal ducts and the nasoethmoid complex is then reduced (Figure 7-14). In certain cases it may be possible to directly wire the nasal and frontal bones and provide satisfactory support (inset).

Excellent results have been achieved using an external fixation device (Figure 7-15). Drill holes, followed by screws, are placed through the outer table of the skull at a point 1 cm medial to the temporal line and 1 cm above the supraorbital rim. An elevator is used to support the nasal complex while a hole is drilled in one of the nasal fragments. A screw is carefully placed through this hole.

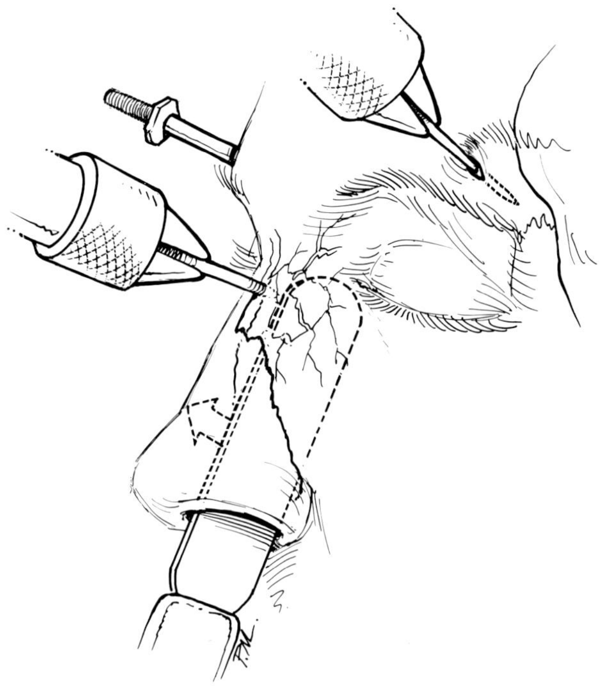

Figure 7-15

A methylmethacrylate bar is then placed on the screws, and the fracture is held in the reduced position until the bar hardens (Figure 7-16). The frontal sinus is then obliterated in the usual fashion. The appliance is left in place for approximately 6 weeks.

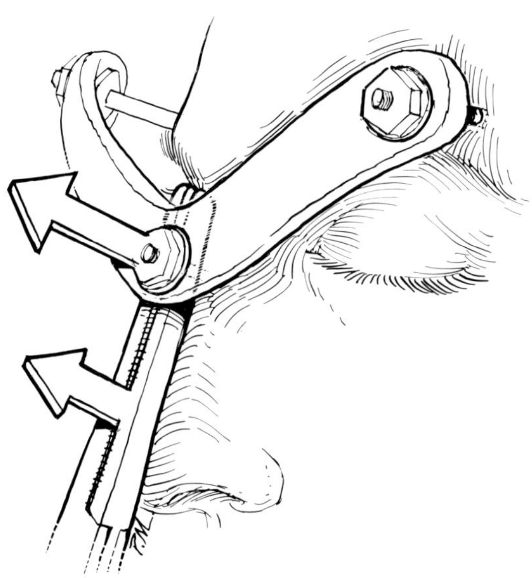

Figure 7-16

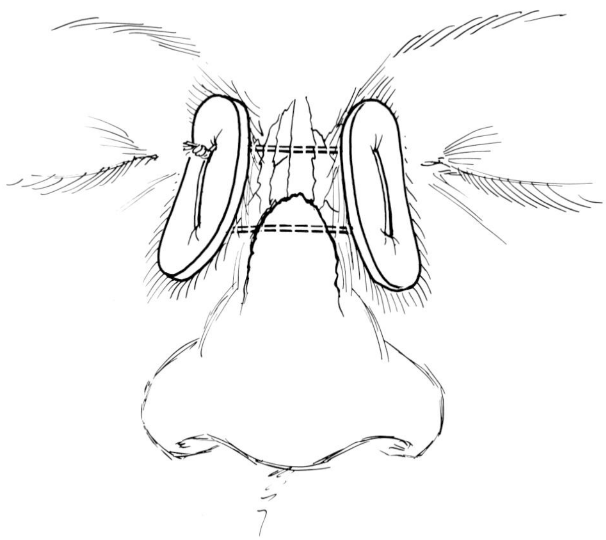

Figure 7-17

ALTERNATIVE TECHNIQUES

Another technique used for stabilizing nasofrontoethmoid fractures is to pass wires through Silastic plates and then through the nasal bones (Figure 7-17). This has not in the author's experience led to completely satisfactory results, particularly in severe fractures.

REFERENCES

1. LeFort, P.: Étude Expérimental sur les Fractures de la Machoire Supérieure. Rev. Chir., 23:479–507, 1901.
2. Mathog, R. H. and Bauer, W.: Posttraumatic Pseudohypertelorism (Telecanthus). *Arch. Otolaryngol.* 105:81–85, 1979.
3. Stranc, M. F. and Robertson, G. A.: A Classification of Internal Injuries of the Nasal Skeleton. *Ann. Plast. Surg.*, 2:468–474, 1979.
4. Williamson, L. K., Miller, R. H., and Sessions, R. B.: Treatment of Nasofrontal Ethmoidal Complex Fractures. *Otolaryngol. Head Neck Surg.*, 89:587–593, 1981.

8

Cerebrospinal Fluid Rhinorrhea

K. J. Lee

Cerebrospinal fluid (CSF) rhinorrhea is a frequent complication of severe facial fractures. Fortunately, CSF rhinorrhea ceases spontaneously without surgical intervention in most cases. Conservative measures such as elevation of the patient's head and mild dehydration may be of value. Serial lumbar punctures or placement of a temporary subarachnoid drainage tube may also stop the drainage. In most cases, observation and conservative measures should be attempted for several days prior to surgical intervention.

It is important to determine the site of the CSF leak. In cases of facial fractures, the frontal sinus and cribriform plate are the most likely areas for leakage. However, if the patient has suffered a temporal bone fracture and the tympanic membrane is intact, then CSF drainage into the middle ear may pass through the eustachian tube and appear as rhinorrhea; obviously, a temporal CSF leak requires a special approach.

SUBLABIAL TRANSSEPTAL TRANSSPHENOIDAL APPROACH

The positioning of the operating table is shown in Figure 8-1. Slight elevation of the operative field above the heart provides better hemostasis, slight hyperextension of the neck affords better visualiza-

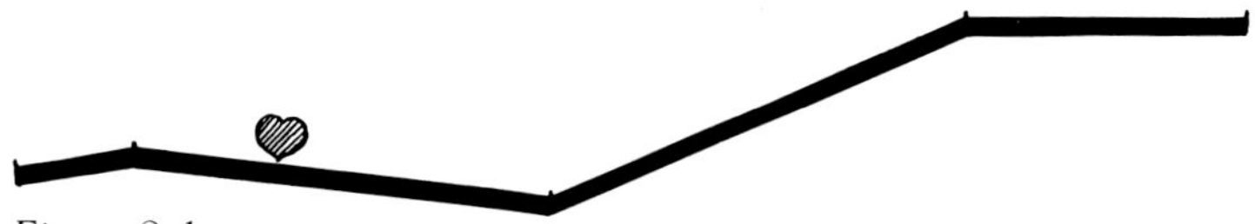

Figure 8-1

tion, elevation of the lower extremities prevents pooling of blood to avoid hypotension, and flexion of the knee provides patient comfort. The patient and the surgeon are positioned so that the operation is performed as if it were a right otologic case. This places the surgeon in the most comfortable posture. An operating microscope with an angled eyepiece and 400-mm lens is used.

After induction of general anesthesia, the operative field is infiltrated with 9 ml 1% lidocaine with epinephrine 1:100,000. Cotton applicators dusted with 300 mg of cocaine flakes are introduced as in a routine rhinoplasty to decongest the nasal mucosa and to achieve further hemostasis. Excellent hemostasis is mandatory in this procedure. Sufficient time should elapse between the infiltration and the first incision. Special attention is given to draping to avoid placing metallic towel clips in the path of a lateral or anteroposterior x-ray to be taken intraoperatively.

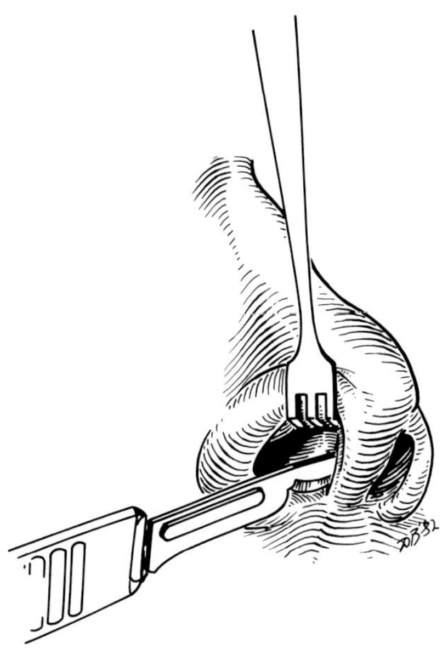

Figure 8-2

The hemitransfixion incision is made in the usual fashion (Figure 8-2). Elevation of the right mucoperichondrium tunnel is started.

The sublabial incision is made with an electric cutting bovie set at No. 2 on the Valley Laboratory SS E2-K machine (Figure 8-3). Care is taken to be sufficiently clear of the gingiva and to leave a cuff of mucosa on the gingiva side for ease of closure. This incision transects the nerve endings of the superior labial branch of the infraorbital nerve, causing temporary anesthesia of the upper lip.

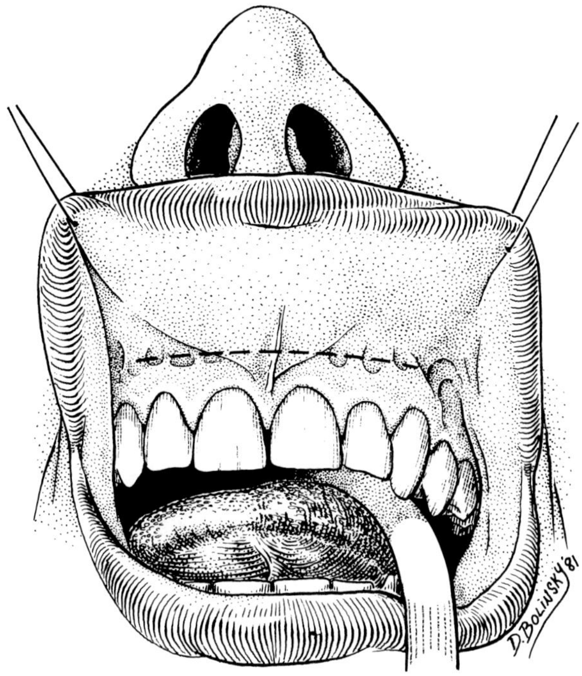

Figure 8-3

The right pyriform aperture is identified, and the mucous membrane is elevated with a Cottle or a McKenty elevator, creating an "inferior tunnel" (Figure 8-4).

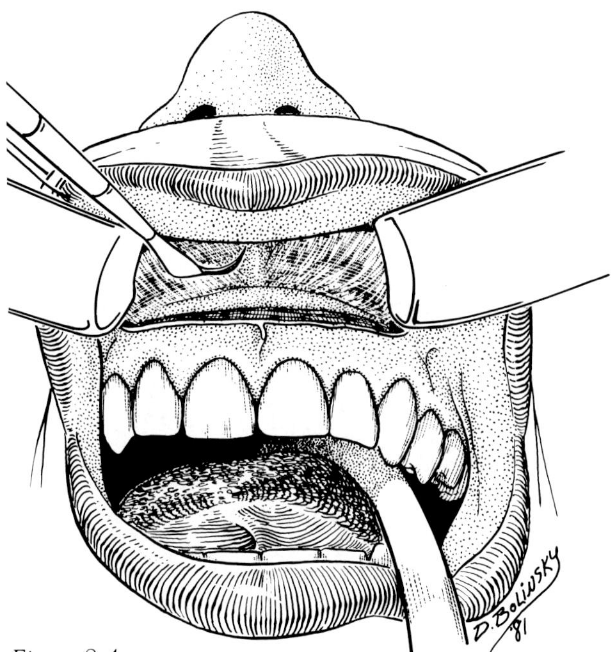

Figure 8-4

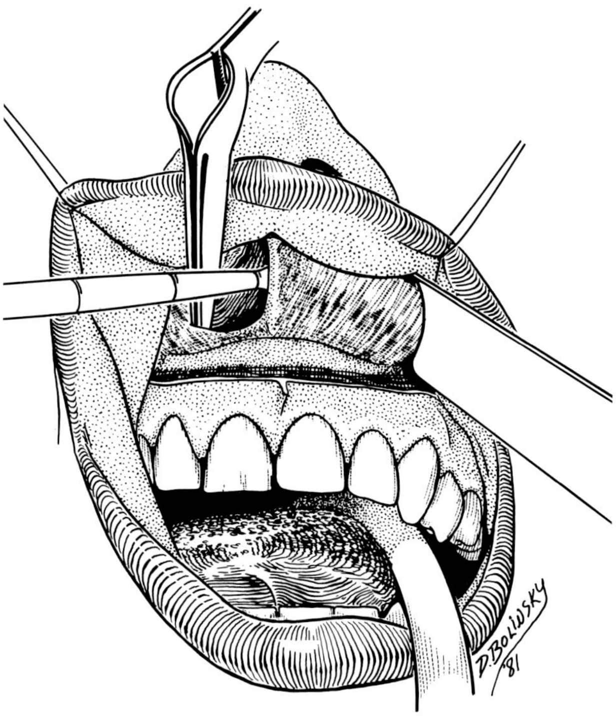

Figure 8-5

The caudal aspect of the septum is identified. The right mucoperichondrium flap is elevated with a Cottle elevator (Figure 8-5). This is connected to the previously made hemitransfixion incision. A Freer septal D knife is used to connect the inferior tunnel to the right mucoperichondrium flap. These decussating fibers can be quite adherent. Careful dissection is needed to prevent a perforation at this juncture. The elevation of the mucoperichondrium flap is carried past the perpendicular plate of the ethmoid on the right.

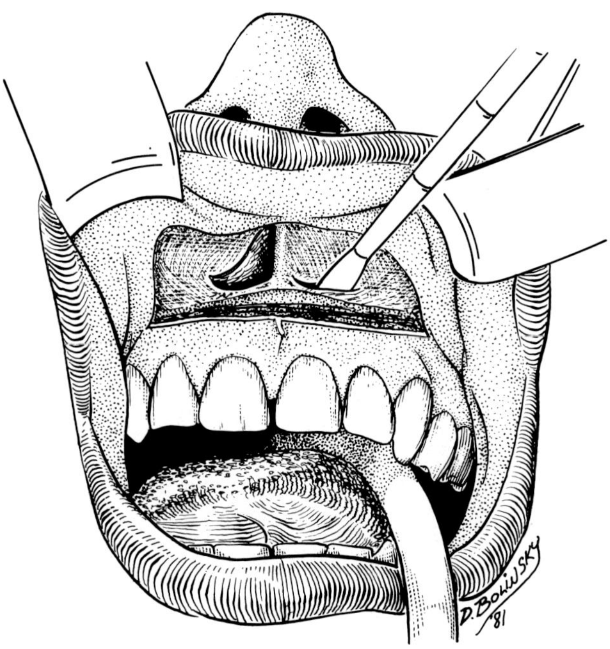

Figure 8-6

The left inferior tunnel is made with a Cottle elevator or a McKenty elevator (Figure 8-6). The decussating fibers are similarly elevated as in the right side, but the full septomucoperichondrium flap is not elevated on the left side of the septum. Leaving the left septomucoperichondrium flap intact would afford a fresh operative approach should one need to return for further repair of recurrent or persistent leaks.

The anterior nasal spine is removed with a rongeur (Figure 8-7).

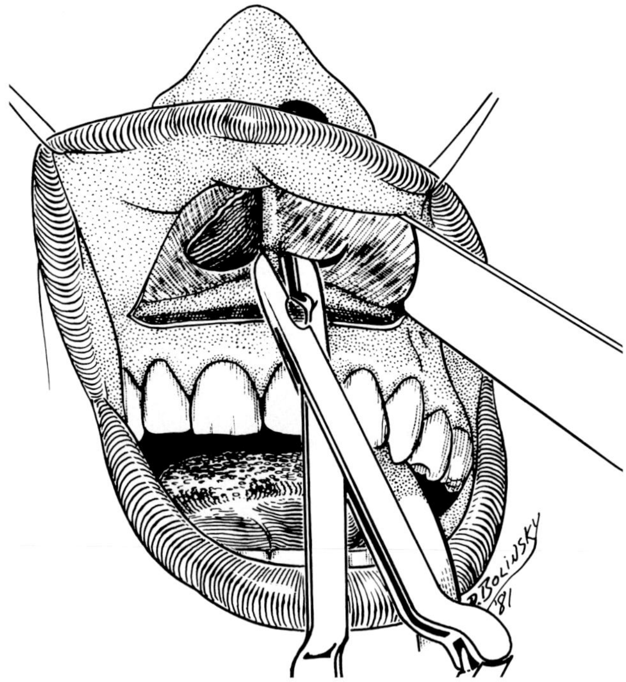

Figure 8-7

With a Lee-Stryker mastoid drill, the pyriform apertures are widened and lowered to better accommodate the self-retaining hypophysectomy speculum (Figure 8-8). The opening of the self-retaining speculum blades is limited by the width of the pyriform apertures anteriorly, and by the midportion of the medial pterygoid plates posteriorly. Care is taken to avoid fracturing the pyriform aperture, the medial pterygoid plates, the medial walls of the orbit, and the medial walls of the maxillary sinuses. Once past the pyriform aperture, the distance between the medial pterygoid plates is the narrowest width in the path of this self-retaining speculum.

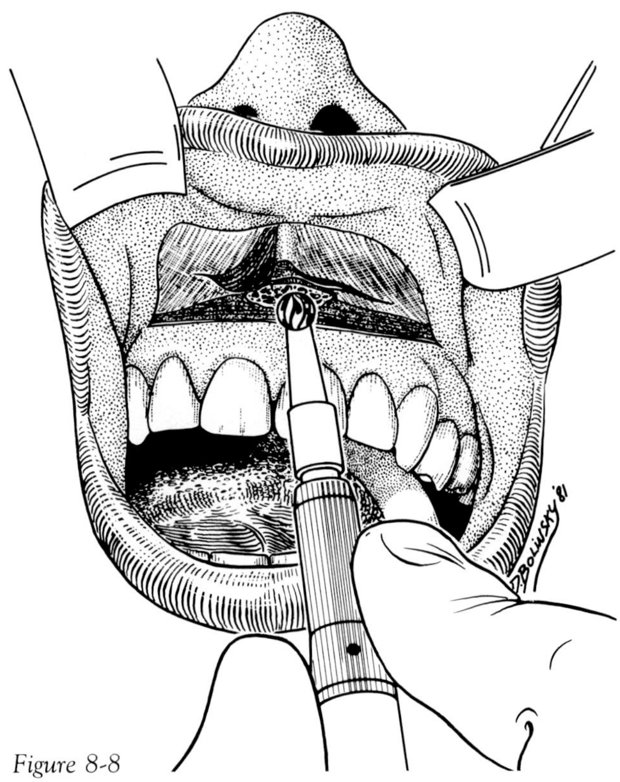

Figure 8-8

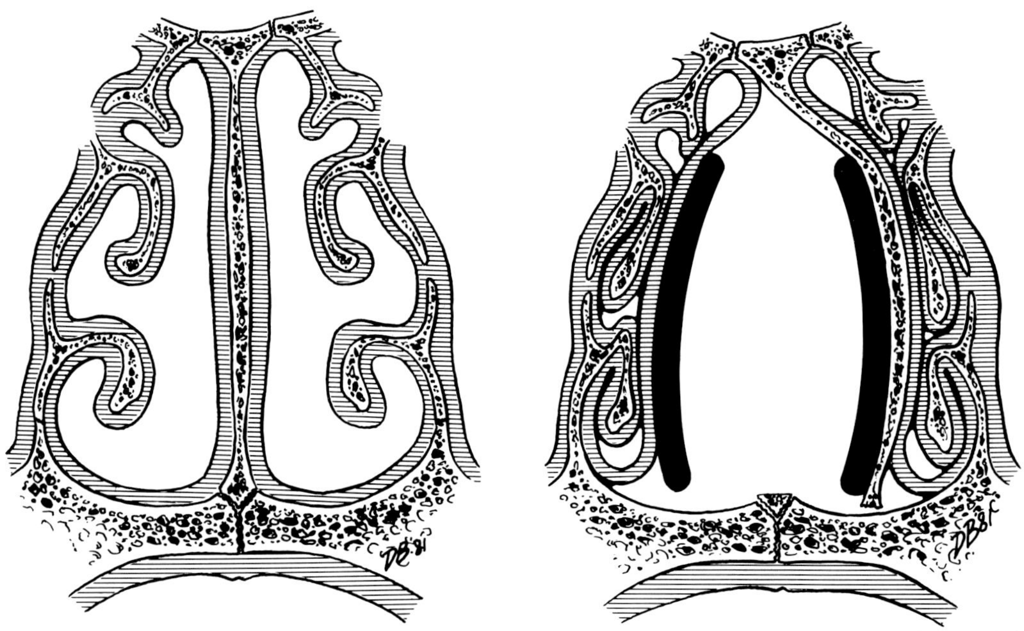

Figure 8-9

The cartilaginous septum is carefully dislocated to the left, carrying with it the intact left mucoperichondrium. The periosteum of the osseous septum (perpendicular plate of the ethmoid) is carefully elevated bilaterally. The osseous septum is removed with a Ferris-Smith forceps, exposing the sphenoid rostrum. It is important to stay in the midline, using the vomer as a guide. The Lee hypophysectomy self-retaining retractor or speculum (or the Hubbard self-retaining retractor) is introduced with the blades in position as shown in Figure 8-9.

With the speculum in place, the anterior wall of the sphenoid sinus between the sphenoid ostia is first removed with Hajek or Kerrison rongeurs (Figure 8-10). Once the sinus is entered, the opening can be carefully enlarged so as to avoid vital structures—including a branch of the sphenopalatine artery, which is located on the inferior aspect of the sphenoid rostrum. The scale on the Lee self-retaining speculum aids in determining the width of the opening at the ends of the blades. Most surgeons need the maximum safe opening permitted by the distance between the two medial pterygoid plates. In most patients this distance is between 2.4 and 2.9 cm.

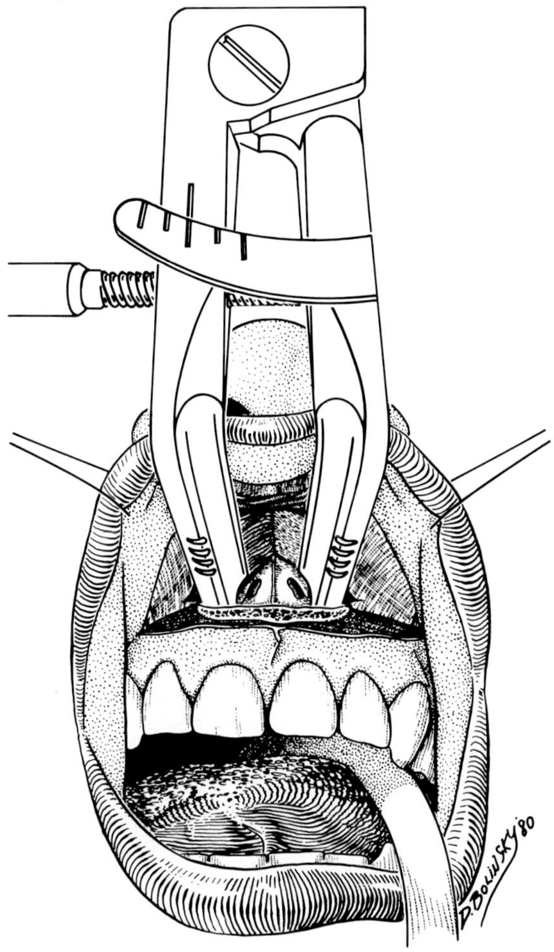

Figure 8-10

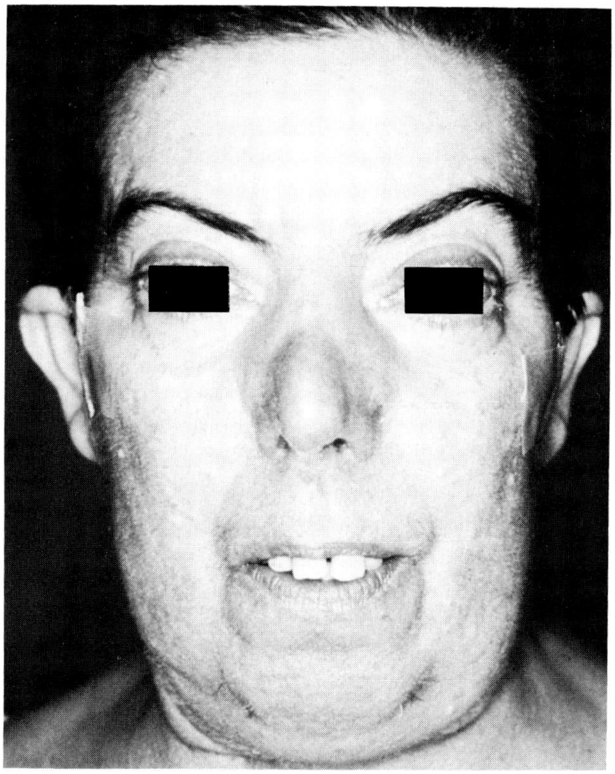

Figure 8-11A

In acromegalic patients or in malformed individuals, the distance between the medial pterygoid plates can be extrapolated by obtaining an x-ray film of the patient with surface metallic markers taped to the skin overlying the temporozygomatic suture line:

$$a'b' = (x'y'/xy) \times ab$$

where $a'b'$ is the actual distance between the medial pterygoid plates, $x'y'$ is the actual distance between the metallic markers that can be measured on the patient, xy is the distance between the metallic markers measured on the x-ray film, and ab is the distance between the medial pterygoid plates measured on the x-ray film (Figure 8-11A and B).

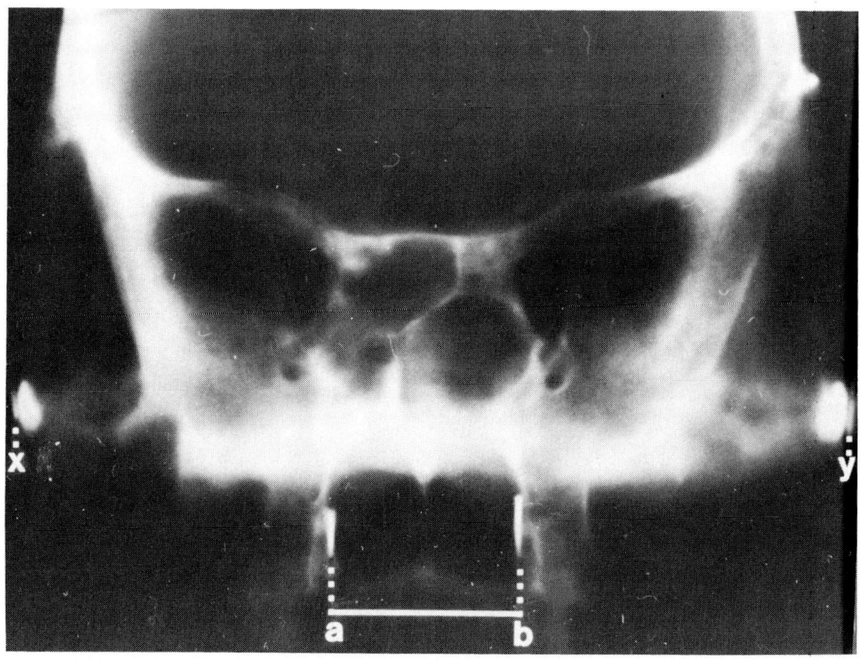

Figure 8-11B

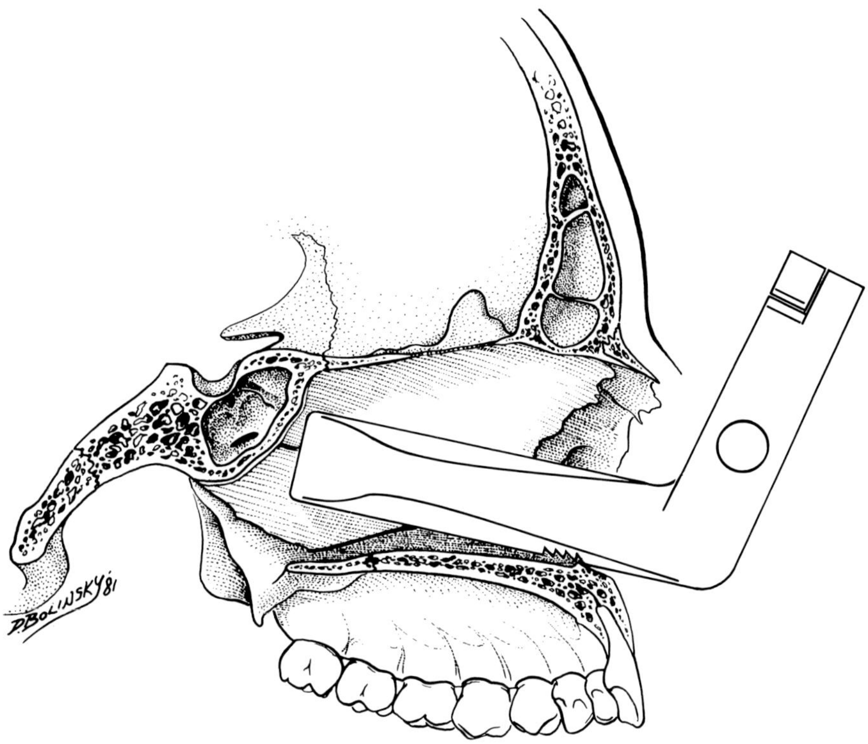

Figure 8-12

Note that if the pyriform aperture and the region of the anterior nasal spine were not previously (Figure 8-8) lowered sufficiently, the speculum blades may now lead the surgeon inferior to the sella. After proper positioning of the self-retaining speculum directing toward the sellar region, the sphenoid is widely exposed (Figure 8-12); the mucosa of the sphenoid sinus is stripped and removed carefully and gently to prevent bleeding. Any slight oozing can be controlled by bipolar electrocautery as well as packing with Surgicel.

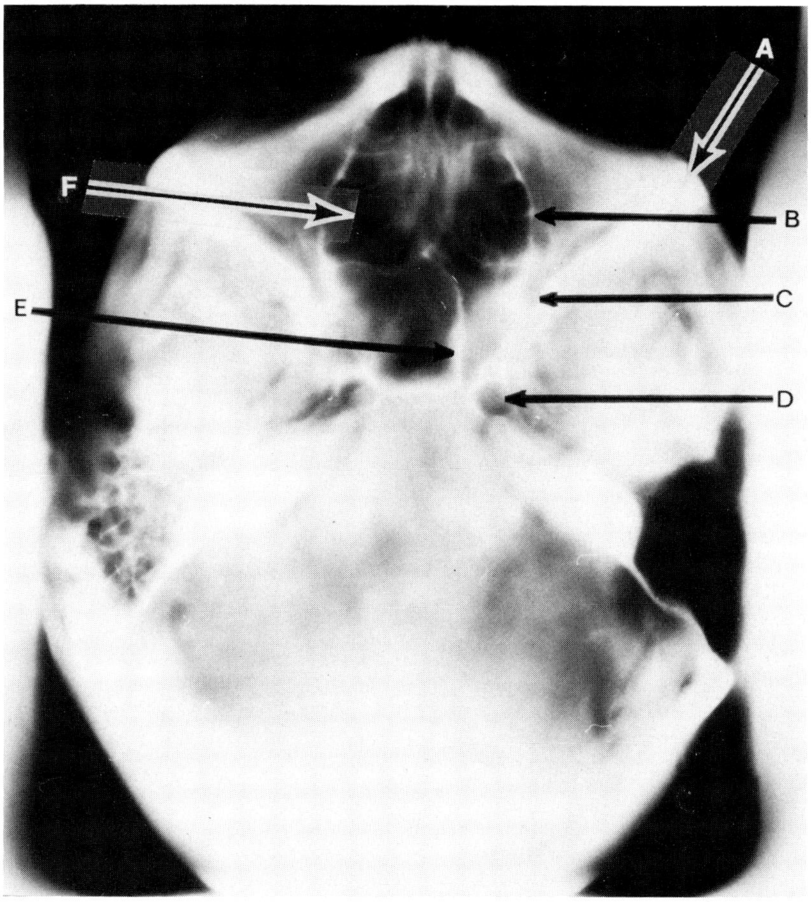

Figure 8-13

The intersphenoid septum is a poor midline landmark. In reviewing 100 consecutive routine sinus x-ray films, Lee[1] found that 34 percent of the patients had a deviated intersphenoidal septum; the deviated intersphenoidal septum may lead the surgeon astray into the carotid canal or cavernous sinus. Hence, it is important to obtain a preoperative submentointersphenoidal laminogram to determine the exact position of the intersphenoidal septum. An example is shown in Figure 8-13, which reveals the following structures: (A) zygoma, (B) lamina papyracea, (C) superior orbital fissure, (D) carotid artery, (E) intersphenoidal septum, (F) posterior ethmoid cells.

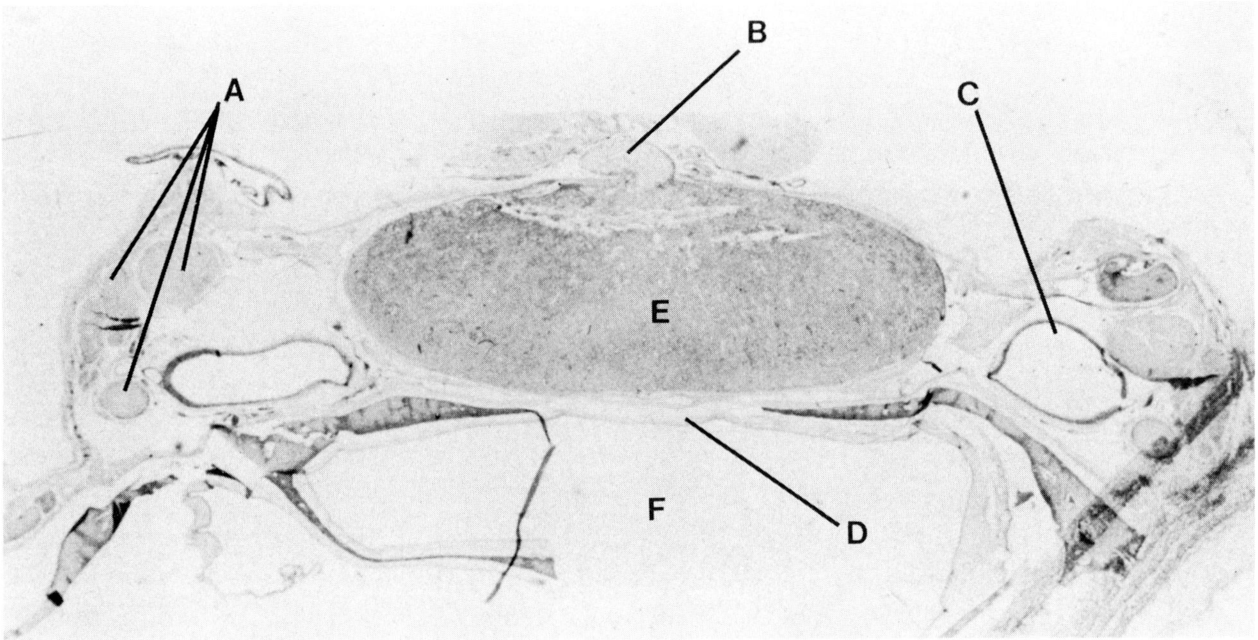

Figure 8-14A

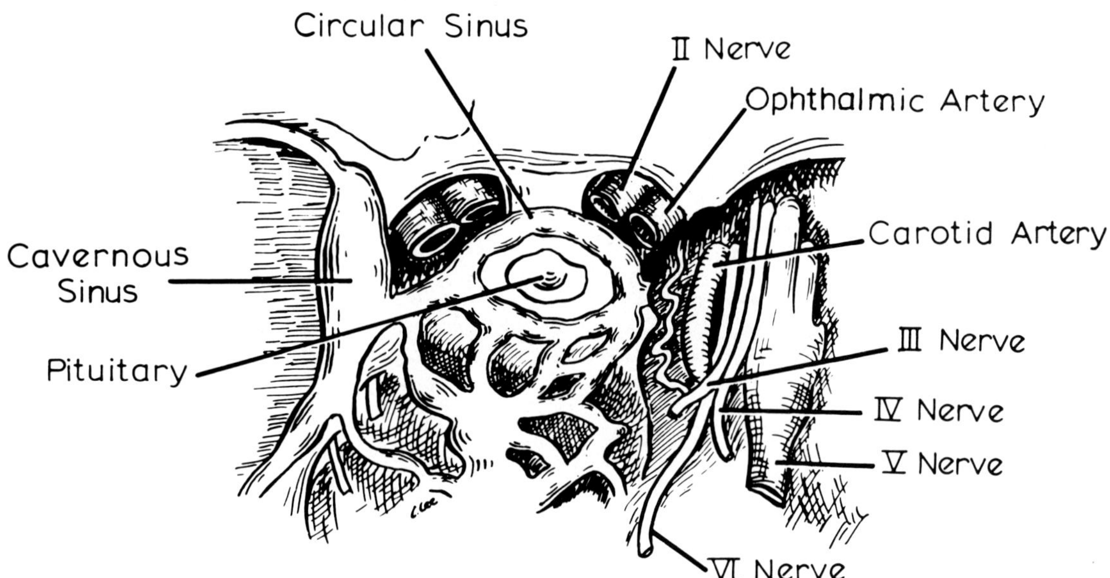

Figure 8-14B

Certain vital structures surrounding the sella are shown in Figure 8-14A and B, including (A) cranial nerves III, IV, V, VI, (B) pituitary stalk, (C) carotid artery, (D) circular sinus (intercavernous sinus), (E) pituitary gland, (F) sphenoid sinus.

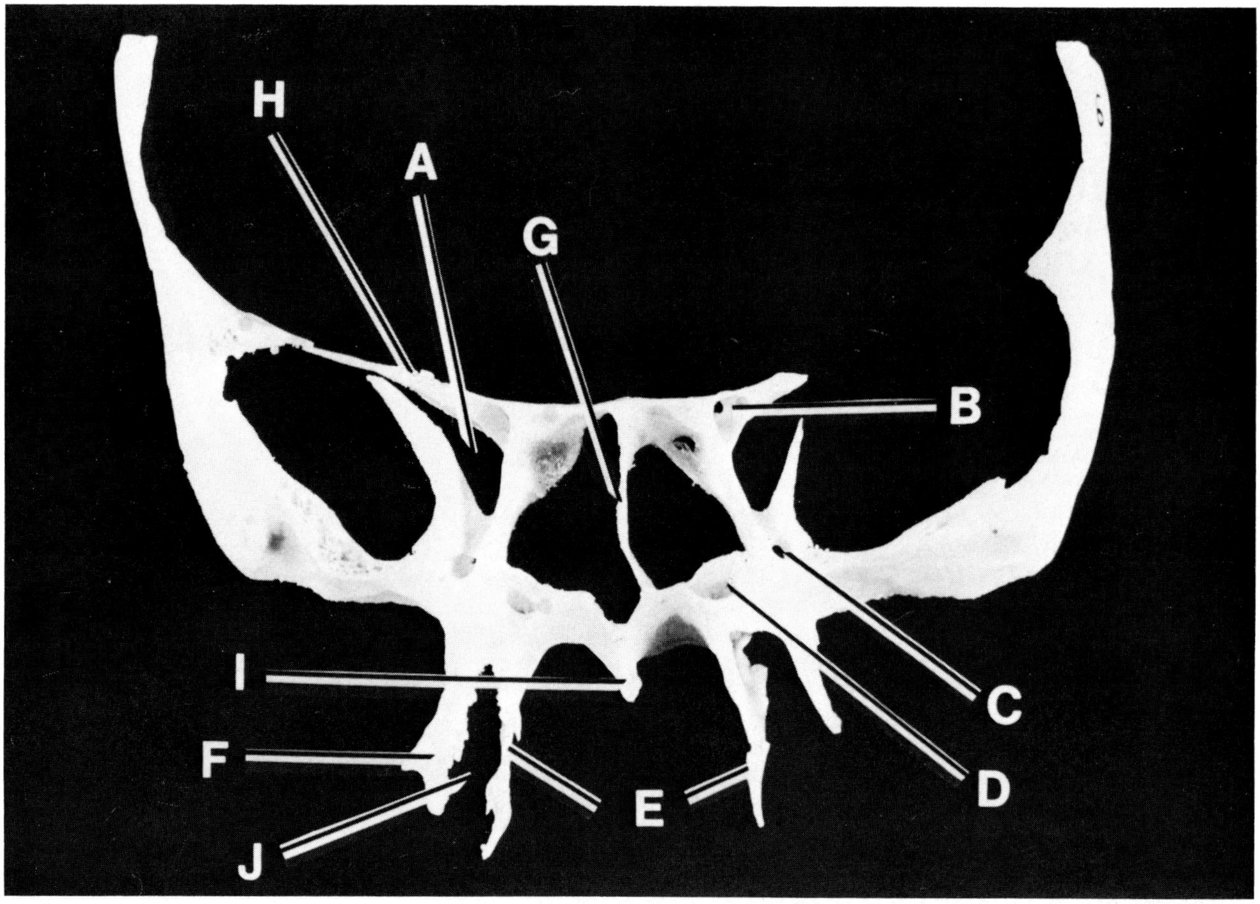

Figure 8-15

In Figure 8-15 certain important anatomic landmarks are shown on a cross section of a dry skull: (A) superior orbital fissure, (B) optic canal, (C) foramen rotundum, (D) pterygoid canal, (E) medial pterygoid plates, (F) lateral pterygoid plates, (G) intersphenoidal septum, (H) lesser wing of sphenoid, (I) sphenoid rostrum, (J) pterygoid fossa.

After the leak is identified, the edges are gently freshened and the fascia that was removed from the upper right thigh (see below) is carefully placed against the leak. In recurrent and persistent CSF leaks, tissue adhesive can be used to glue the fascia in position in addition to using packing. The sphenoid cavity is packed with adipose connective tissue, care being taken that the mucosa of the sphenoid has been completely removed. Hemostasis is achieved with surgicel and/or pressure by neuropledgets and bipolar cautery. A tight or snug packing is required. The self-retaining speculum is carefully retracted and the nasal cavities are packed swiftly. A strip of Telfa (2 cm × 7 cm) is placed against the septum on both sides and Nu-gauze impregnated with bacitracin ointment is packed snugly in the nasal cavities as in a routine septoplasty or septorhinoplasty. If there is any laceration in the mucosa, care is taken not to invert or evert the edges. Two septal-columella mattress sutures (3-0 chromic) are placed to close the hemitransfixion incision. The sublabial incision is closed with interrupted 3-0 chromic simple stitches. It is important to have the nasal packing ready prior to removing the self-retaining speculum to avoid unnecessary bleeding and movement of the adipose tissue packing in the sphenoid sinus. (Prior to use, the fascia and adipose connective tissue harvested from the upper right thigh are bathed in a solution of streptomycin, 50 mg in 1000 ml normal saline, or in a solution of bacitracin, 100,000 units in 1000 ml normal saline.)

Subsequently, the nose is taped in the usual fashion and the sublabial region is kept clean with mouth irrigation using 150 mg clindamycin (Cleocin) and 250 ml saline. This is done three times a day. If the patient is allergic to clindamycin, a warm saline rinse may suffice. The patient is instructed to refrain from physical exertion as well as from stooping forward. The patient is kept in the semi-Fowler position for 72 hours postoperatively and is advised to keep the head of the bed elevated for the next 2 weeks. The nasal packing is removed in 7 days. Postoperative antibiotic therapy is advocated for 7 days; the choice of antibiotic is guided by preoperative nasal culture and sensitivity.

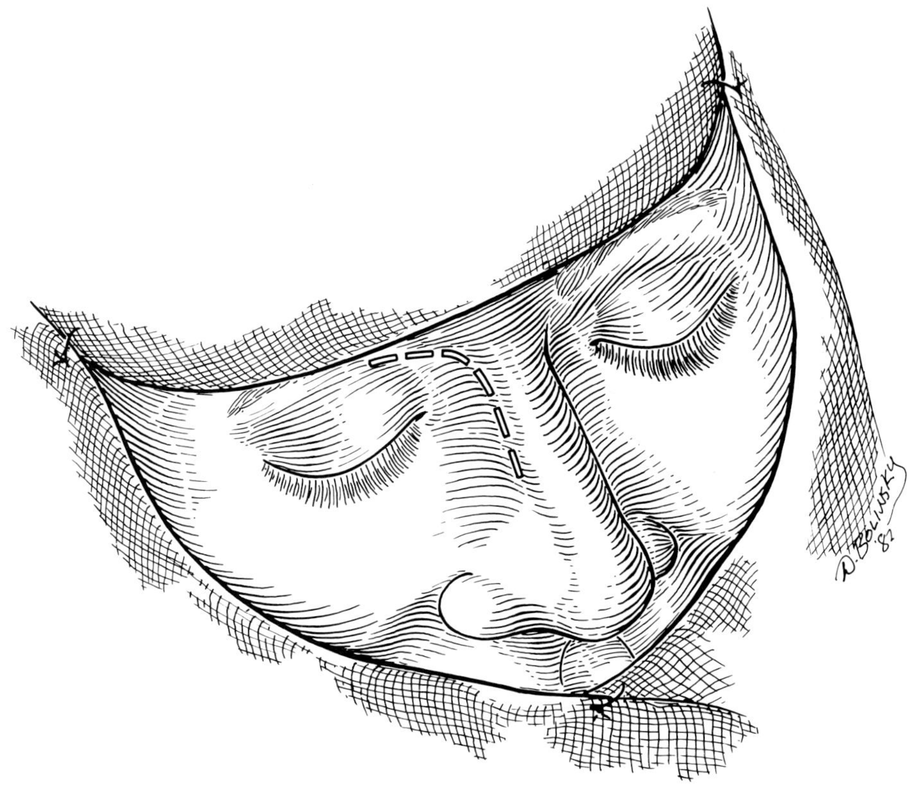

Figure 8-16

TRANSETHMOIDAL APPROACH

The patient is prepared, draped, and positioned as in a routine septorhinoplasty (Figure 8-16). During the draping, it is important to avoid any metallic towel clips so as not to interfere with any intraoperative x-ray films. The incision is made as outlined in Figure 8-17.

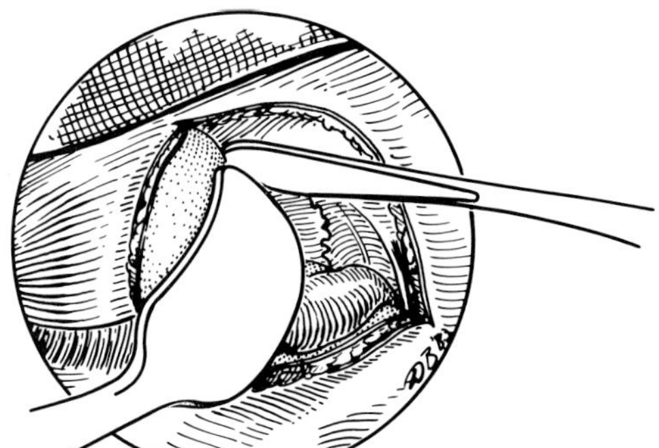

Figure 8-17

Temporary tarsorrhaphy is performed. The ethmoid bone is exposed with the Freer elevator or Cottle elevator, and the orbital contents carefully protected by an orbital retractor (Figure 8-17). When retracting the orbit, it is important not to apply too much and too constant a pressure.

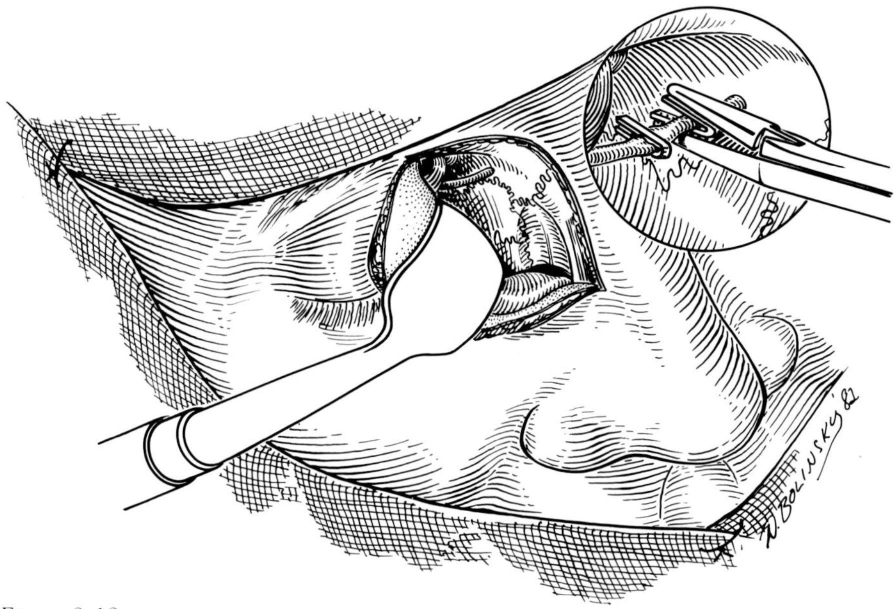

Figure 8-18

The lacrimal fossa is identified as well as the anterior ethmoidal artery, which is cross-clipped with hemoclips and transected (Figure 8-18).

The anterior ethmoid sinus is opened with bone curettes (Figure 8-19).

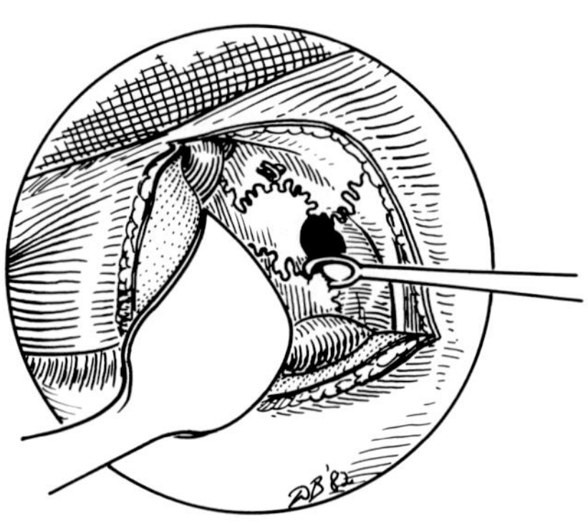

Figure 8-19

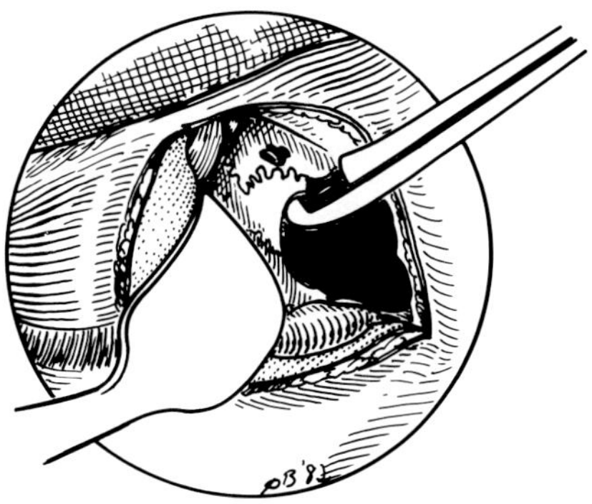

Figure 8-20

With Kerrison rongeurs, the area is widened to allow access to the anterior and posterior ethmoidal sinuses (Figure 8-20).

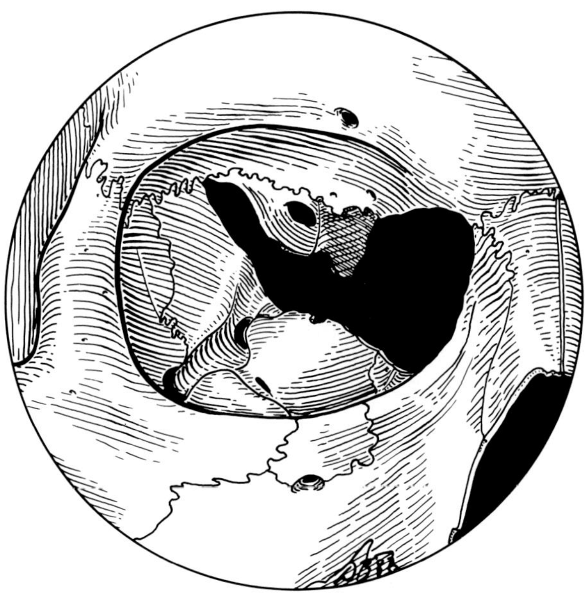

Figure 8-21

Through this approach, the sphenoid sinus is encountered and entered, exposing the sella turcica (Figure 8-21). The mucosa of the sphenoid sinus is stripped.

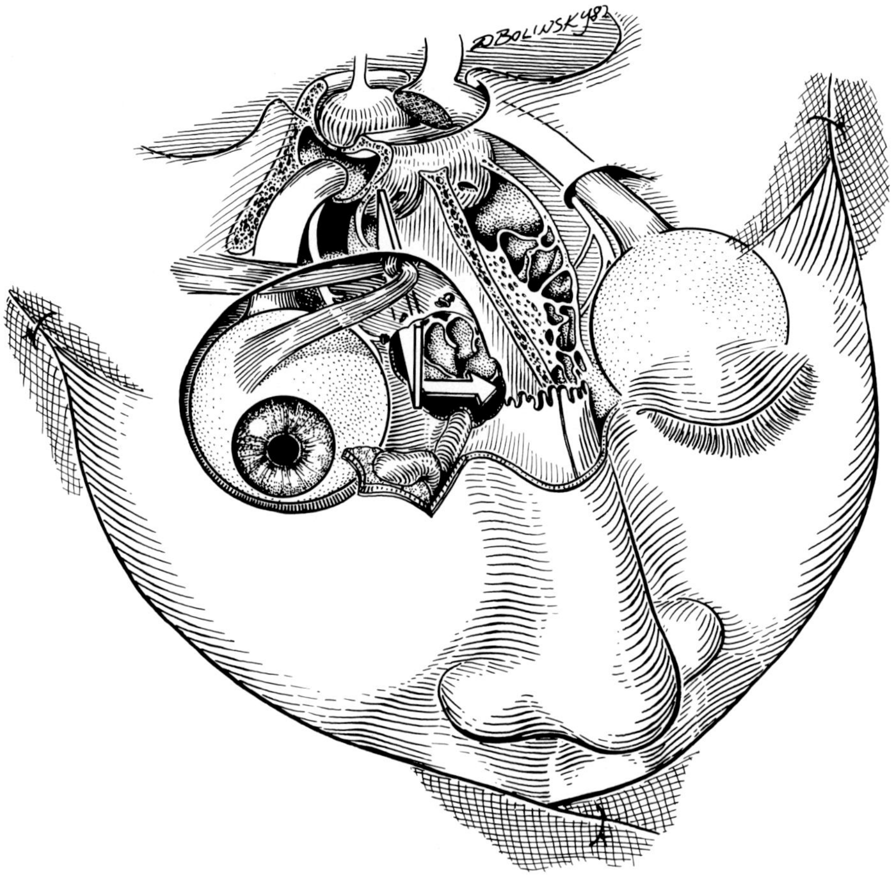

Figure 8-22

The path taken in the transethmoidal transsphenoidal approach to the sella is shown in Figure 8-22.

After the leak is identified, the edges are gently freshened. The fascia taken from the upper right thigh is placed over the leak and the sphenoid sinus is packed with adipose connective tissues. Care is taken to ascertain that all the mucosa of the sphenoid sinus had been removed. Surgicel packing is used in the sphenoid and ethmoid sinus regions to control some troublesome oozing. A Cottle speculum is used to visualize through the nasal cavity to inspect the operative site. Surgicel packing may be introduced through the nasal cavity to further close the surgical wound intranasally. Occasionally, small amounts of Nu-gauze impregnated with bacitracin ointment may be necessary for nasal packing for 2–3 days. (Prior to use, the fascia and adipose connective tissue harvested from the upper right thigh are bathed in a solution of streptomycin, 50 mg in 1000 ml normal saline or in a solution of bacitracin, 100,000 units in 1000 ml normal saline.)

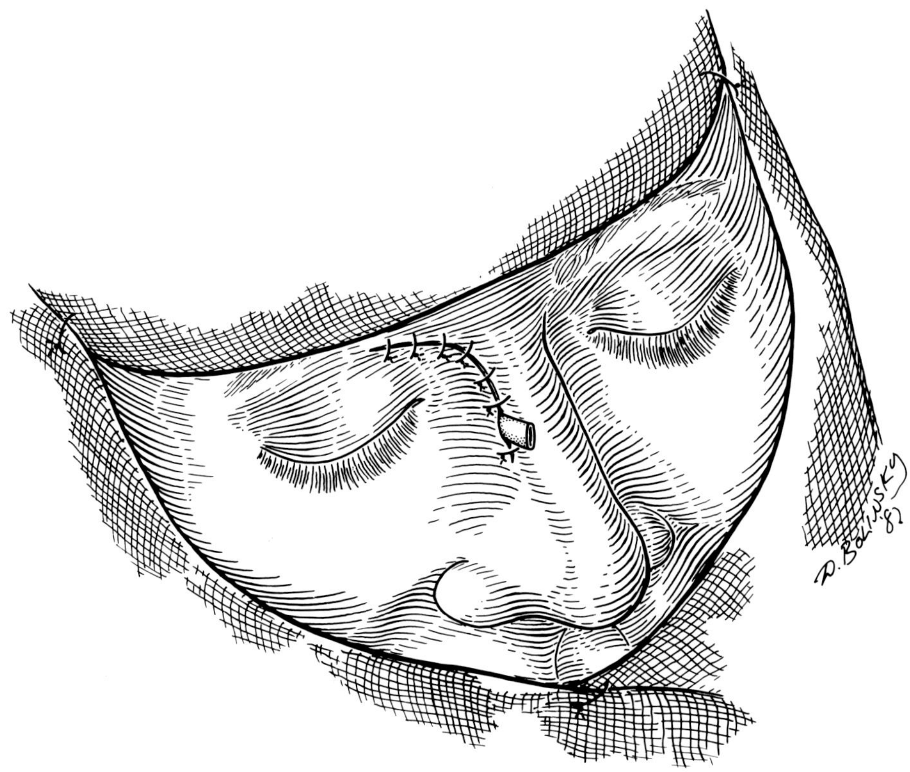

Figure 8-23

The incision is closed with interrupted 3-0 chromic sutures and interrupted 5-0 nylon sutures with a small rubber drain in position (Figure 8-23). The temporary tarsorrhaphy sutures are removed and eye pads are used to form a gentle pressure dressing. Postoperative treatment is the same as for the sublabial transseptal transsphenoidal approach.

REFERENCES

1. Lee, K. J.: The Sublabial Transseptal Transsphenoidal Approach to the Hypophysis. *Laryngoscope* 87(suppl. 10): 1–65, 1978.
2. Montgomery, W. W.: Transethmoidosphenoidal Hypophysectomy with Septal Mucosal Flap. *Arch. Otolaryngol.*, 78:68–77, 1963.
3. Sasaki, C. T.: Pituitary Ablation for Carcinoma of the Breast: Transethmoidal Approach to the Sella. *Otolaryngol. Clin. North Am.*, 14:391–404, 1981.

9

Laryngeal and Tracheal Trauma

OPEN REPAIR OF LARYNGEAL INJURY

Direct laryngoscopy and bronchoscopy are performed to assess the degree of laryngeal and tracheal injury (Figure 9-1).

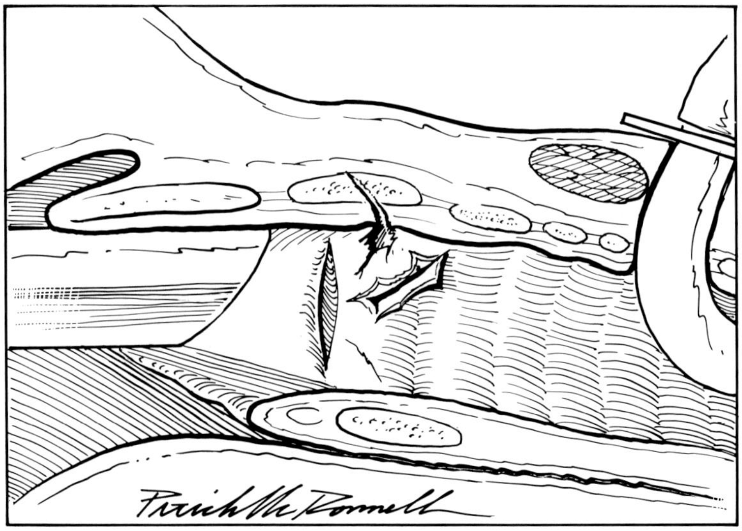

Figure 9-1

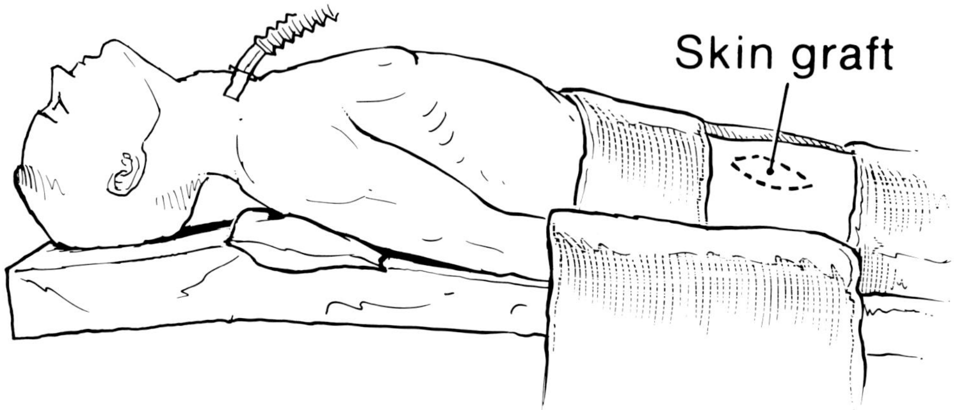

Figure 9-2

The patient is placed in a supine position with the shoulder roll in place to extend the neck (Figure 9-2). The neck as well as the thigh (for a skin graft) are prepared and draped.

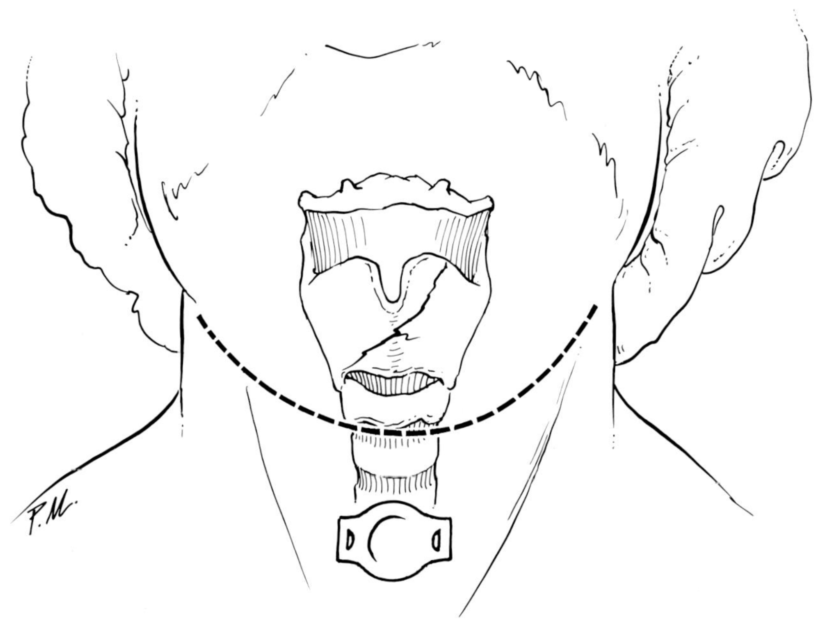

Figure 9-3

A U-shaped incision is made crossing the midline at the level of the cricoid cartilage and flaps are elevated superiorly and inferiorly in a plane deep to the platysma muscle (Figure 9-3). The superior flap is elevated to the level of the hyoid bone.

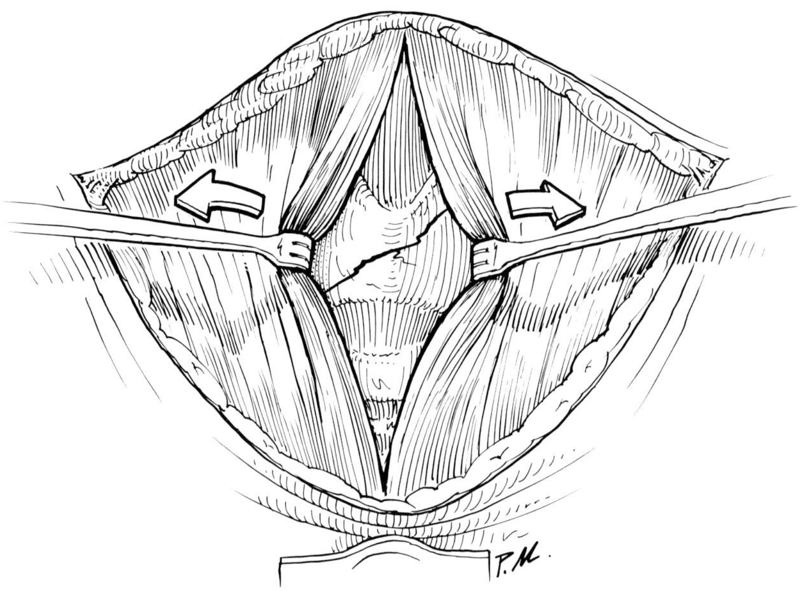

Figure 9-4

The strap muscles are carefully divided in the midline and retracted laterally, exposing the thyroid cartilage (Figure 9-4).

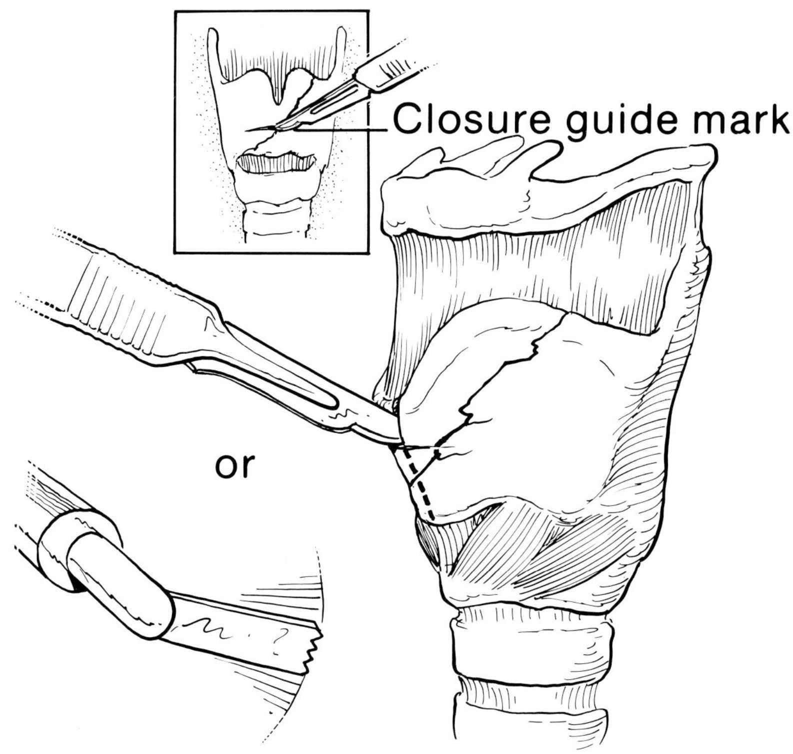

Figure 9-5

A small horizontal mark is made in the thyroid cartilage, which will be important during closure of the laryngofissure (Figure 9-5). A scalpel is used to cut carefully through the midline of the thyroid cartilage. An oscillating saw may be necessary when the thyroid cartilage is calcified.

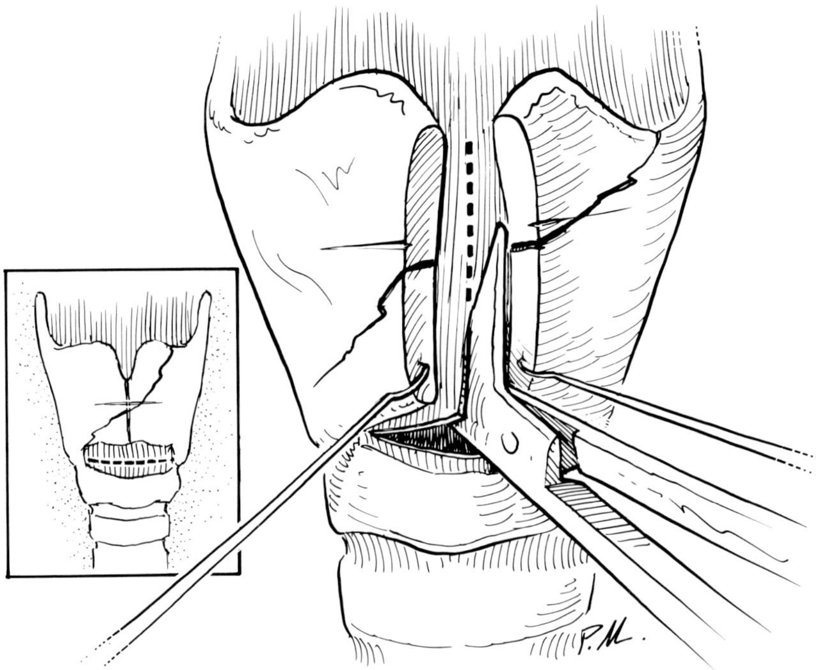

Figure 9-6

A horizontal incision is made in the cricothyroid membrane and, with skin hooks retracting the edges of the transected thyroid cartilage, the incision is extended superiorly under direct visualization (Figure 9-6).

Great care is taken to ensure that the incision passes through the anterior commissure of the true vocal cords and, once superior to this area, extends either to the left or the right to avoid transecting the epiglottis (Figure 9-7).

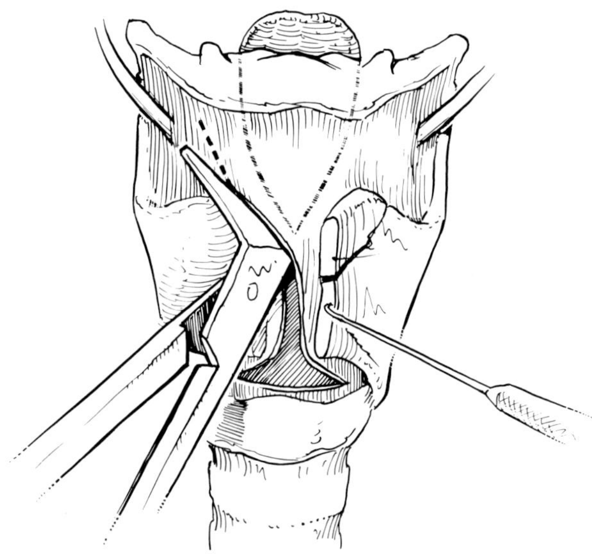

Figure 9-7

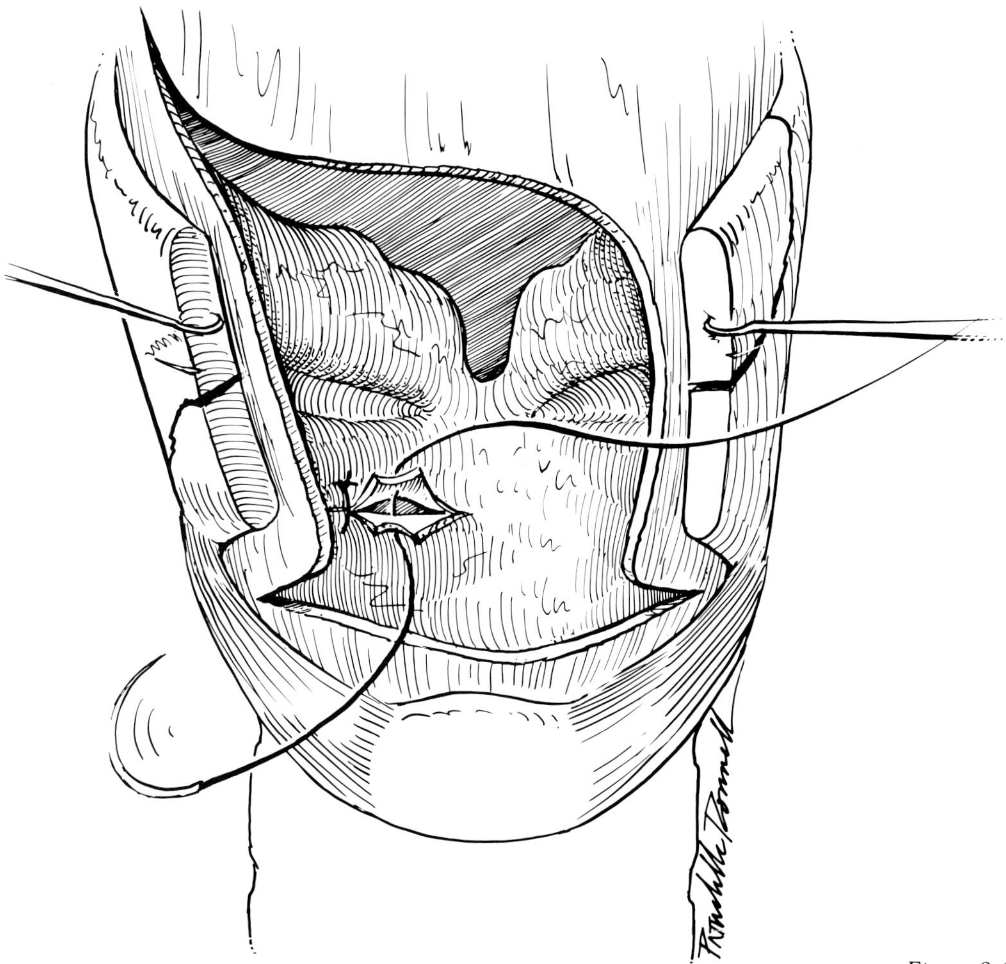

Figure 9-8

All mucosal lacerations are closed with small absorbable sutures (Figure 9-8).

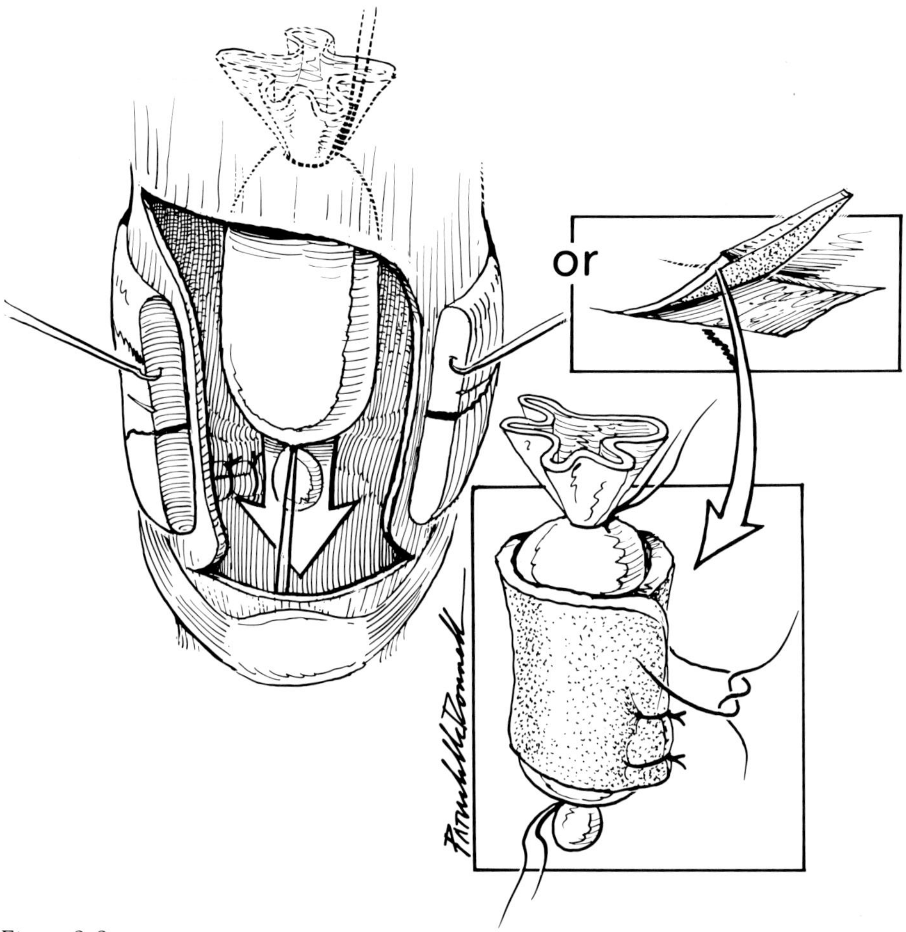

Figure 9-9

A soft laryngeal stent is fabricated from the finger of a surgeon's glove filled with foam latex rubber (Figure 9-9). (See Figure 9-13 for more details on stent fabrication.) In the event of extensive mucosal lacerations a skin graft is sewn around the stent.

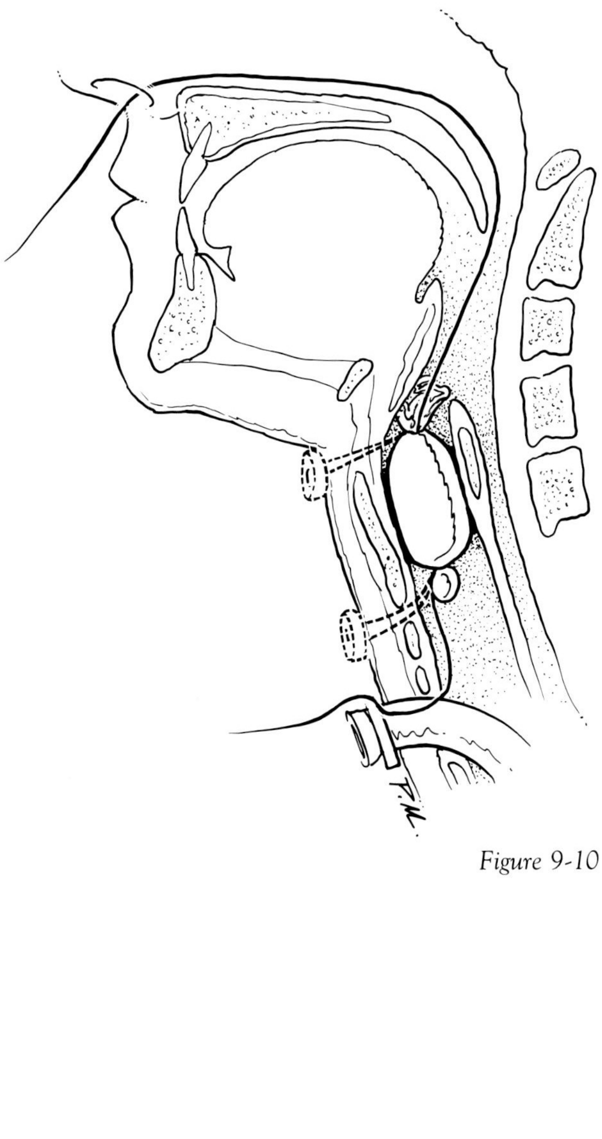

Figure 9-10

The stent is held in place by sutures that pass through the nose and the tracheotomy site (Figure 9-10). Another technique of stabilizing the stent is to place sutures through the thyrohyoid and cricothyroid membranes and tie them over buttons on the neck skin.

The laryngeal fracture is reduced and fixation is obtained with stainless steel wire (Figure 9-11). In the same fashion the laryngofissure is closed; care is taken to match the two halves of the mark on the thyroid cartilage. The incision in the cricothyroid membrane is also closed with absorbable sutures. An absorbable suture passed through the anterior aspect of each cord to the external perichondrium helps prevent the development of an anterior web.

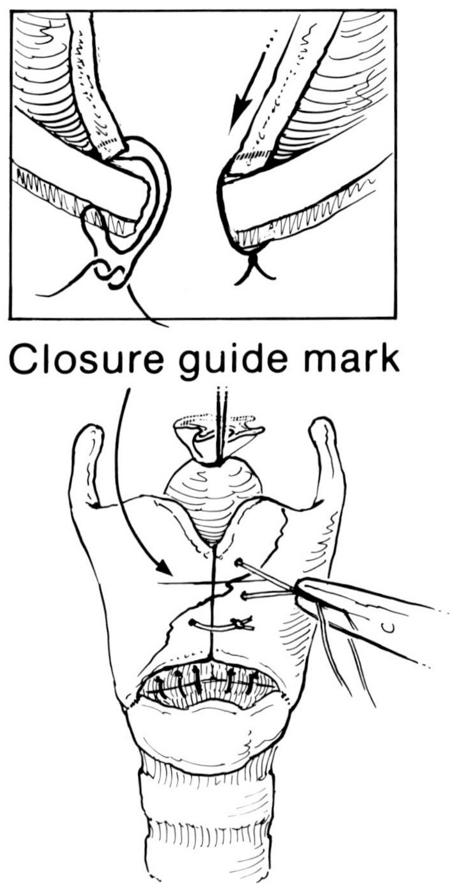

Figure 9-11

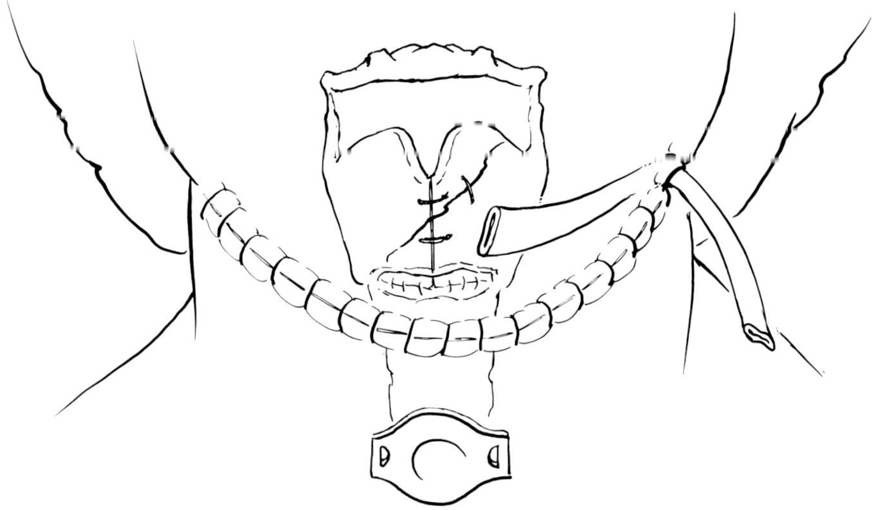

Figure 9-12

The strap muscles are sutured in the midline (Figure 9-12). A Penrose drain is placed between the strap muscles, and the skin flap is closed.

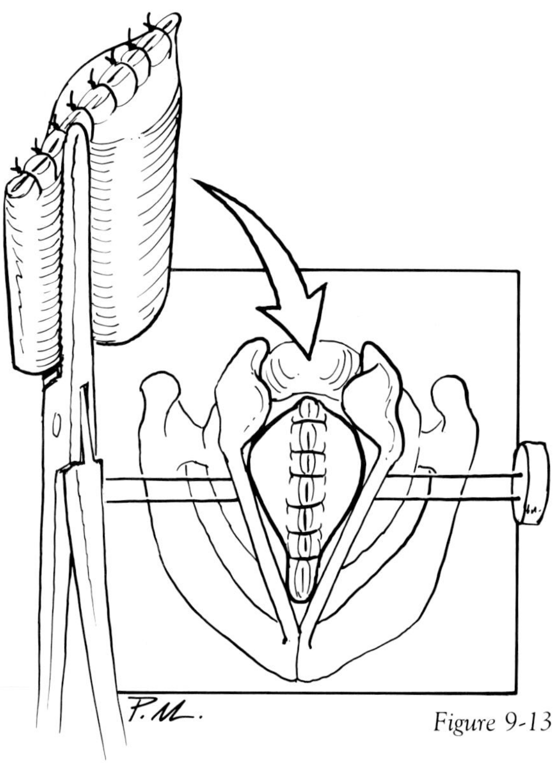

Figure 9-13

SPECIAL TECHNIQUES: STENT FABRICATION

A variety of material has been used for stents. Stents can basically be divided into hard or soft varieties. The sponge-filled surgical glove finger is the most widely used soft laryngeal stent. Prefabricated laryngeal stents are produced by a variety of manufacturers and are generally made from a Silastic block.

An endotracheal tube can be used to make a laryngeal stent (Figure 9-13). A segment of the appropriate-size endotracheal tube is obtained. The superior end of the endotracheal tube is closed with nonabsorbable sutures to prevent aspiration; a clamp can be used to "pinch" one side of the tube. The tube is placed in the autoclave. The clamp can then be removed, and the narrowed area used to maintain the anterior commissure. Stents may be held in place by nonabsorbable sutures passed from the stent through the thyroid cartilage and skin and secured over buttons.

LARYNGEAL AND SUBGLOTTIC STENOSIS

Although many cases of laryngeal and subglottic stenosis can be conservatively managed with serial dilatations, more aggressive therapy is indicated in those patients in whom dilatation is not satisfactory.

A vertical incision is made in the midline in the area of stenosis. Generally the scar tissue is left in place as further mucosal dissection may give rise to even more scar tissue. However, if the amount of scar tissue is quite marked, then a submucosal resection of the scar tissue may be performed. After the length of the stenotic area is determined, an appropriate length of hyoid bone is measured and all of the suprahyoid muscles as well as the infrahyoid muscles on one side are freed from the hyoid bone (Figure 9-14).

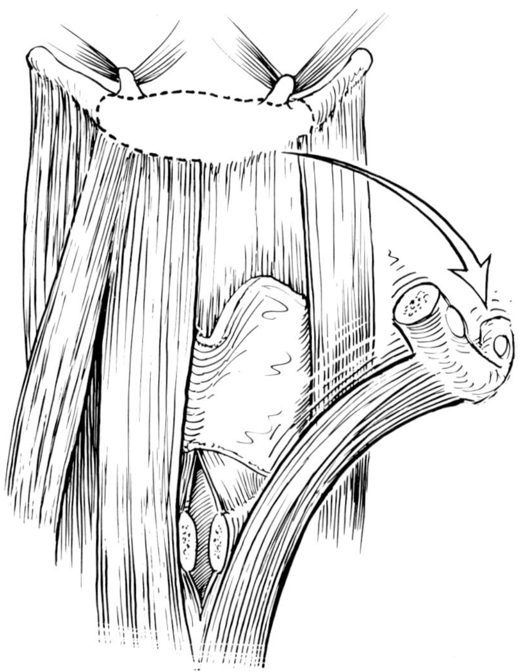

Figure 9-14

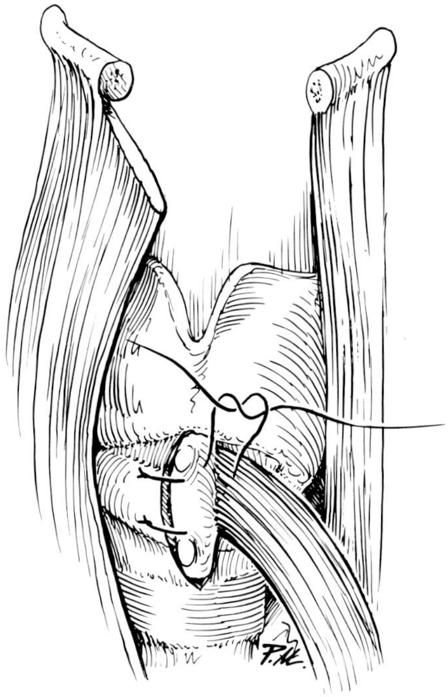

Figure 9-15

After the graft is trimmed so that it fits into the laryngeal incision properly, nonabsorbable sutures are passed through the graft and the surrounding laryngeal cartilages (Figure 9-15). It may be necessary to drill holes in the hyoid bone to pass the sutures. The graft is secured in position. Stenting is optional, although if there has been loss of mucosa, a skin graft should be applied.

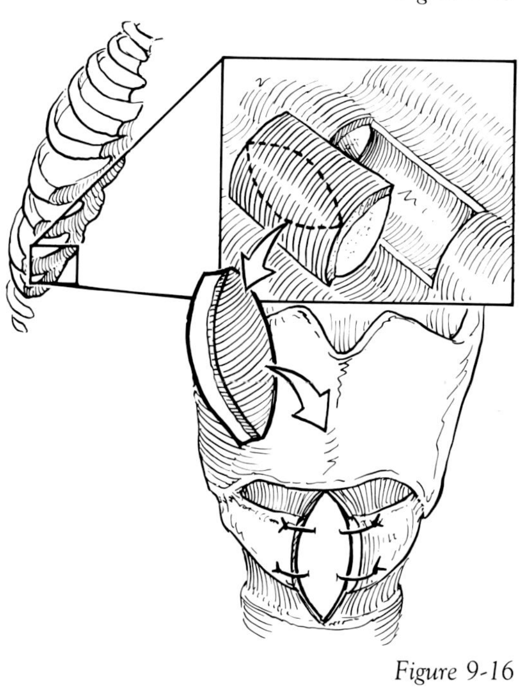

Figure 9-16

ALTERNATIVE TECHNIQUES AND SPECIAL CASES

Excellent success has also been obtained with a costal cartilage graft, which is similarly placed in the laryngeal incision (Figure 9-16).

In order to obtain an adequate airway in cases of severe laryngeal stenosis, the larynx may also be widened posteriorly. Following laryngofissure, an incision is made in the midline through the cricoid cartilage; great care is taken not to penetrate the mucosa just posterior to the cricoid cartilage. A graft of costal cartilage is fashioned so that the edges of the cricoid cartilage fit into the concavely beveled edges of the graft (Figure 9-17). A stent with skin graft is then used to maintain the lumen.

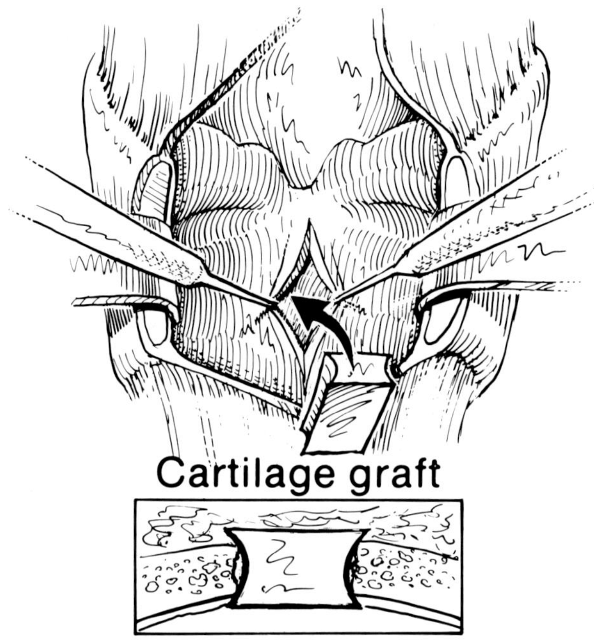

Figure 9-17

OPEN REPAIR OF TRACHEAL INJURY

Primary repair should be attempted in the vast majority of tracheal injuries. Most tracheal injuries can be explored through a U-shaped incision in the lower neck (Figure 9-18).

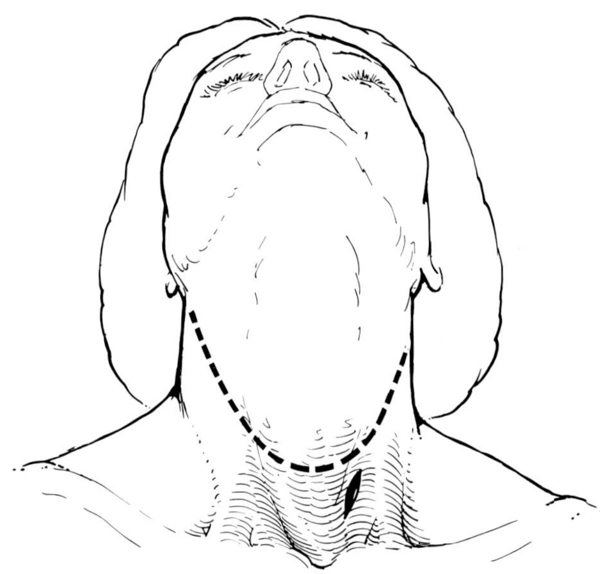

Figure 9-18

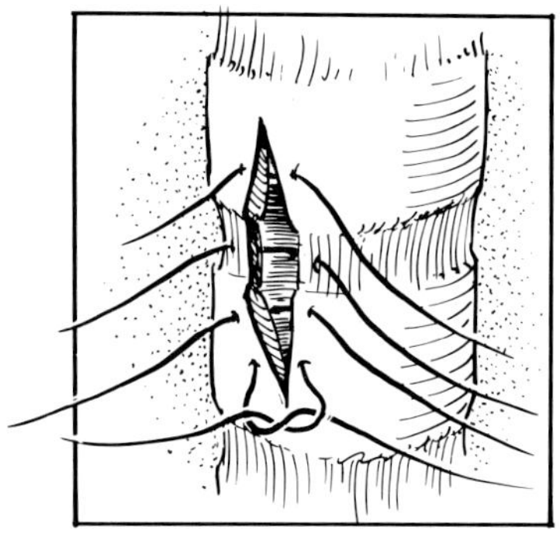

Figure 9-19

Penetrating injuries such as stab wounds can be repaired by using nonabsorbable sutures to close the tracheal perforation with careful approximation of the tracheal cartilages (Figure 9-19).

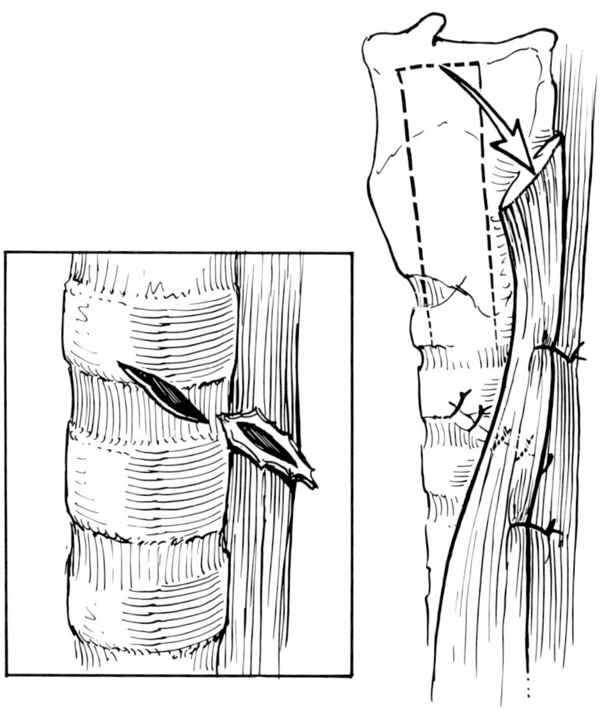

Figure 9-20

If there is a concomitant esophageal injury, rotation of some of the strap muscles to separate the tracheal and esophageal injuries helps prevent the development of a tracheoesophageal fistula (Figure 9-20).

TRACHEAL RESECTION

If stenosis develops following repair of the tracheal injury, it is best repaired with resection and anastomosis. Selected acute tracheal injuries (particularly blast injuries) may also be repaired using this technique. It is generally preferable, however, to attempt a primary repair, and then if stenosis develops, proceed with tracheal resection. This is particularly true when there is a concomitant esophageal injury. The two factors that are most critical to a successful repair are minimal tension on the anastomosis and avoidance of devascularization of the tracheal margins.

The patient is placed on the operating table in a supine position with a shoulder roll in place (Figure 9-21). The neck and chest are prepared and draped.

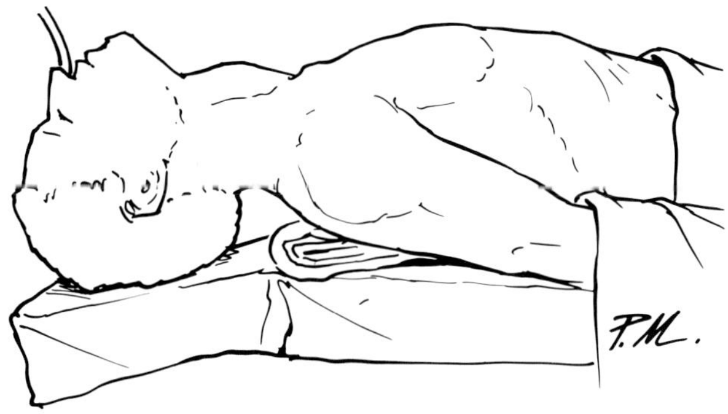

Figure 9-21

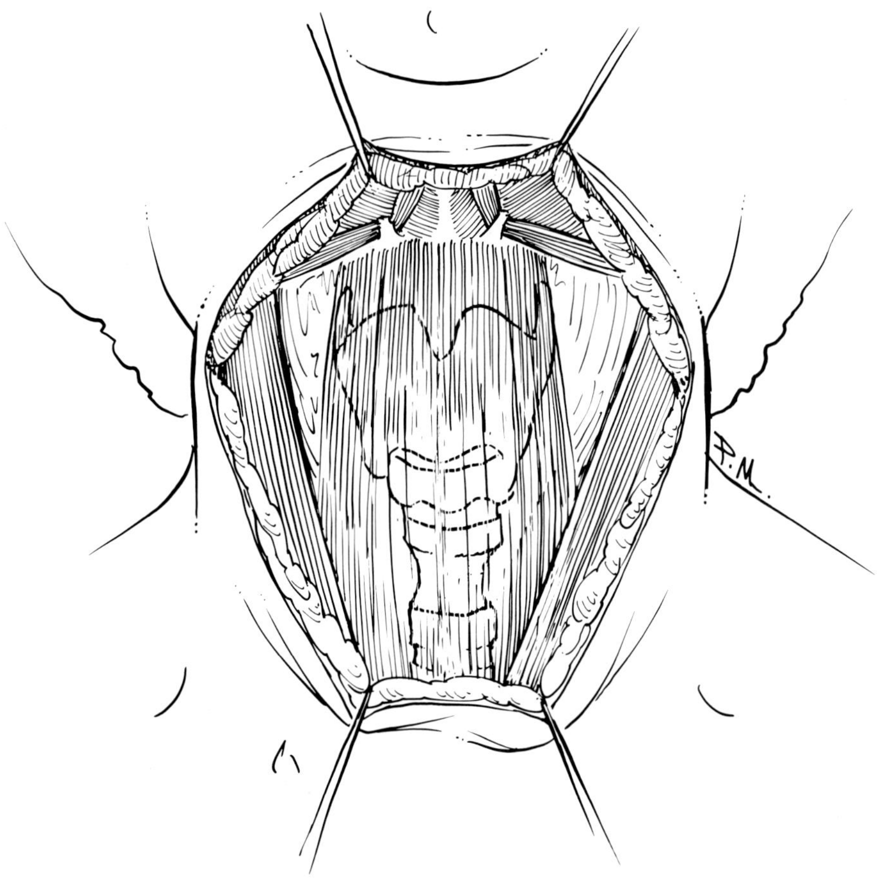

Figure 9-22

A U-shaped incision is made, and flaps are elevated in a plane just deep to the platysma muscle, with the superior flap elevated above the hyoid bone and the inferior flap elevated to the level of the sternal notch (Figure 9-22).

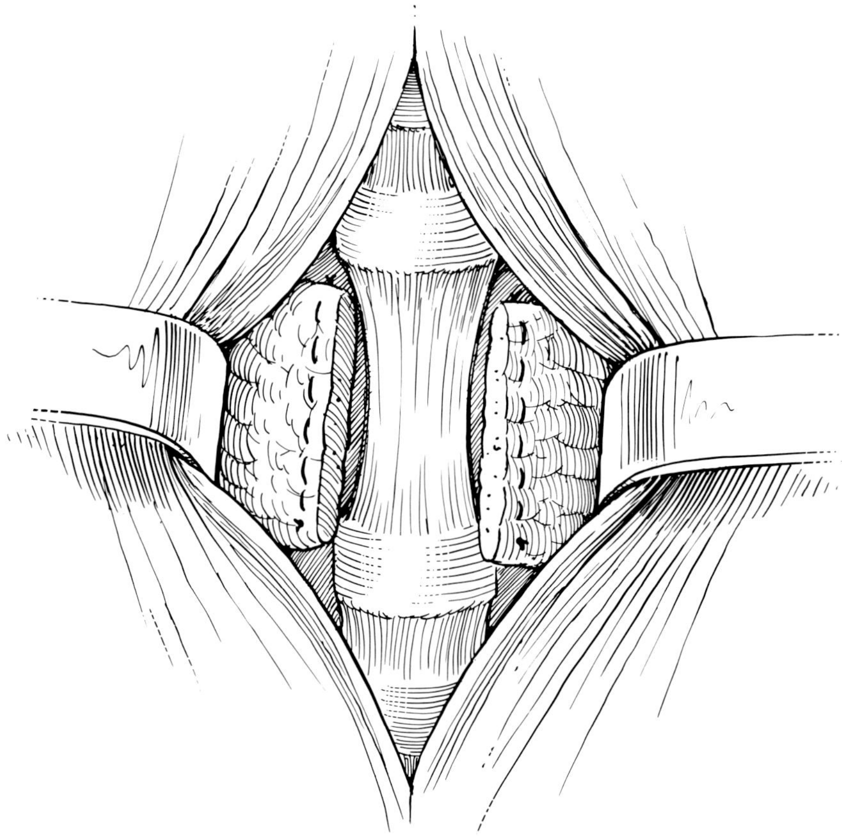

Figure 9-23

The strap muscles are divided in the midline, exposing the laryngeal cartilages and the thyroid gland. The thyroid gland is divided in the midline, and the transected edges are sutured with absorbable suture (Figure 9-23).

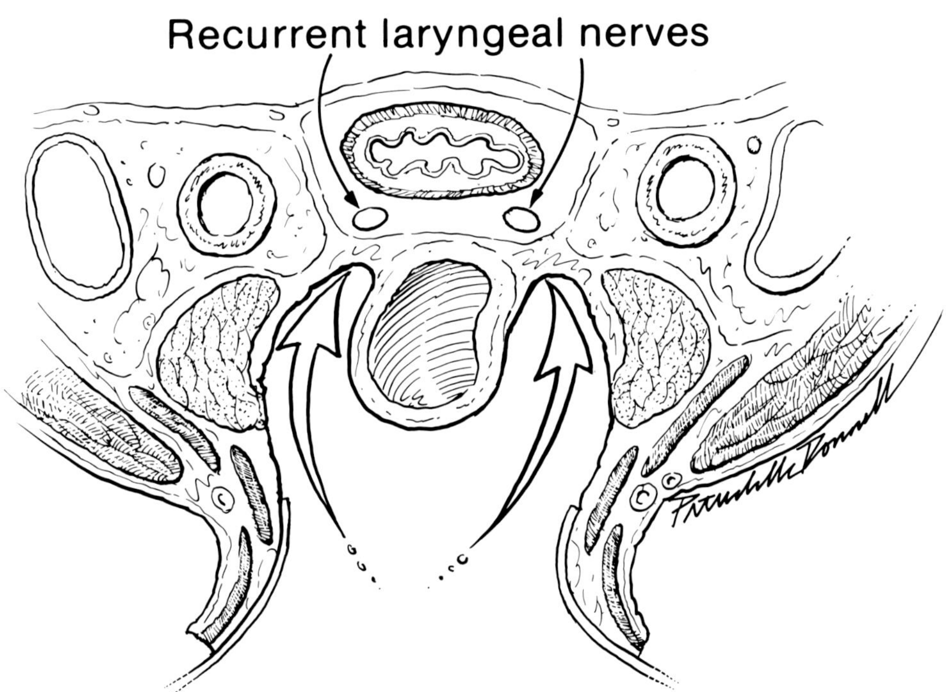

Figure 9-24

The trachea is skeletonized in the area of the stenosis (Figure 9-24). Great care is taken to stay directly on the tracheal cartilage; this prevents damage to the recurrent laryngeal nerves and helps develop the correct plane between the trachea and esophagus.

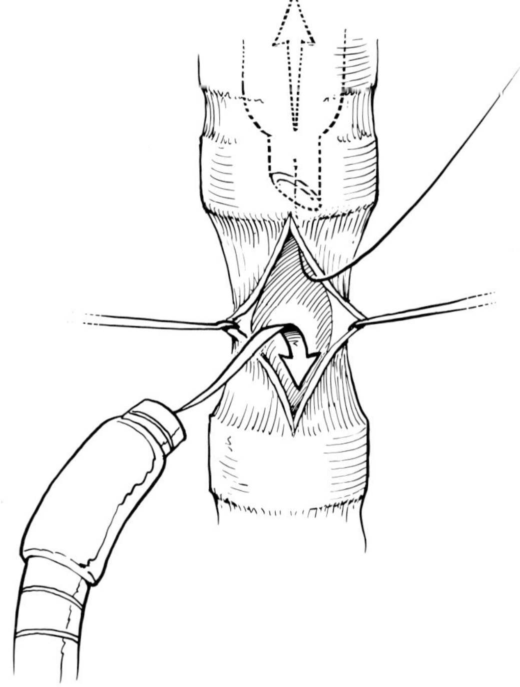

A vertical incision is made in the area of the stenosis. The previously placed endotracheal tube is withdrawn superiorly and an anode-type tube is passed into the tracheal opening (Figure 9-25). A heavy silk suture passed through the end of the withdrawn endotracheal tube facilitates its replacement later.

Figure 9-25

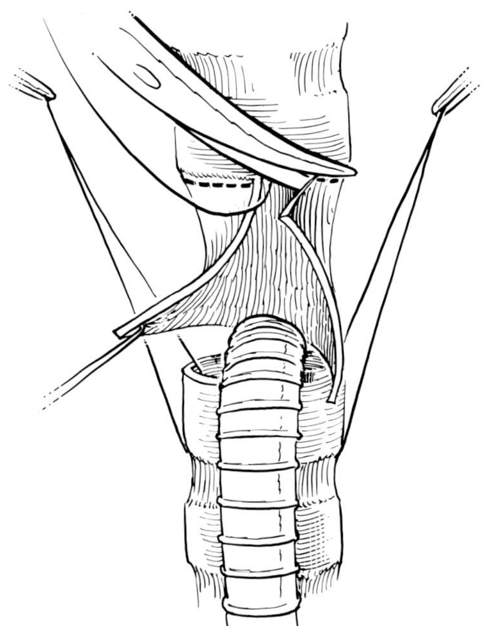

Under direct visualization of the internal aspect of the trachea, the stenotic segment is resected (Figure 9-26). Care must be taken to prevent the thoracic trachea from retracting into the chest; this can be accomplished by placing traction sutures through the trachea.

Figure 9-26

The thoracic trachea is mobilized by blunt dissection in a plane just deep to the pretracheal fascia anteriorly and in the soft tissue plane between the trachea and esophagus posteriorly (Figure 9-27). Care must be taken not to injure the laterally based blood supply to the trachea for more than 1 cm from the margin of resection.

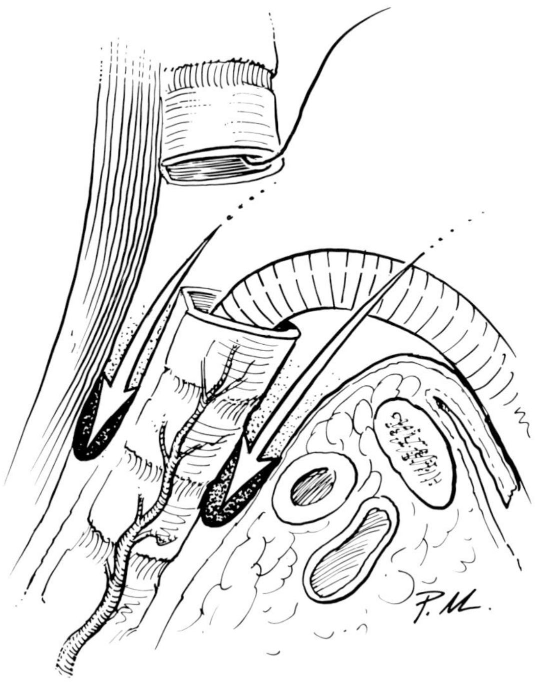

Figure 9-27

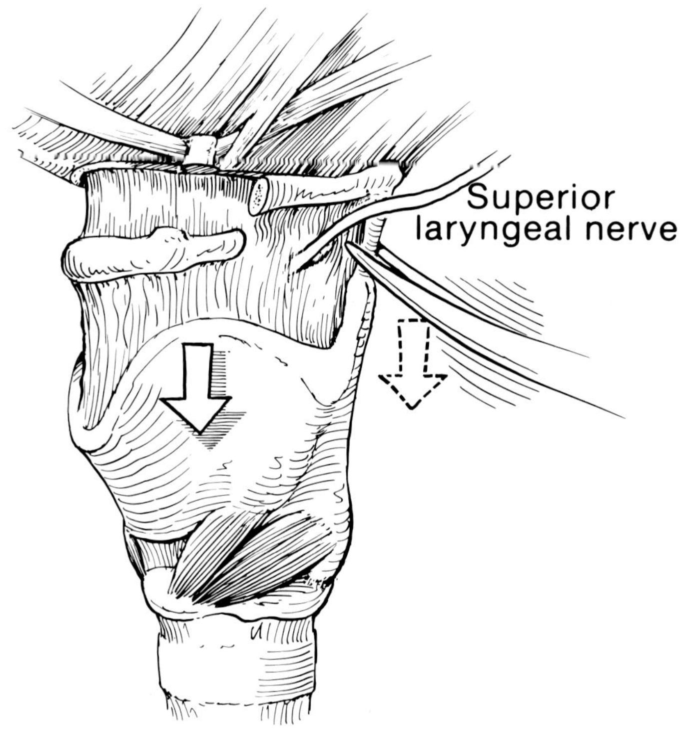

Figure 9-28

A suprahyoid laryngeal release is accomplished by dividing the suprahyoid muscles at the level of the hyoid bone and transecting the greater cornua of the hyoid bone (Figure 9-28). The suspensory ligaments attached to the superior cornua of the thyroid cartilage are also transected. The suprahyoid technique spares the superior laryngeal nerves as well as the supraglottic lymphatics.

Lateral stay sutures are placed through both ends of the trachea, and prolene sutures are placed in the posterior wall such that the knots will be outside the tracheal lumen (Figure 9-29).

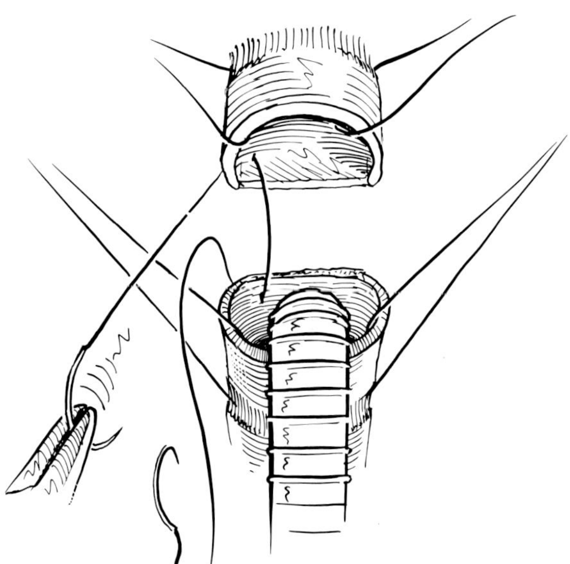

Figure 9-29

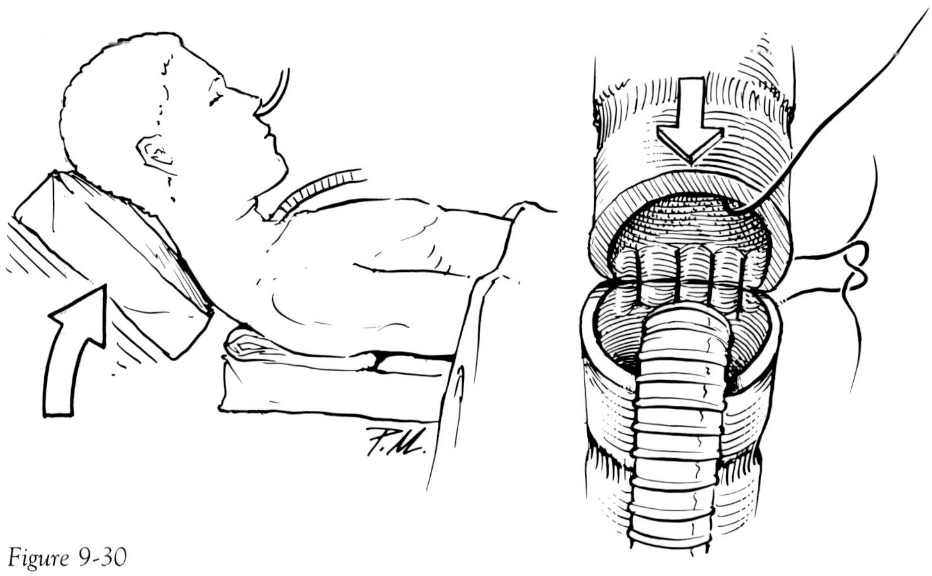

Figure 9-30

The neck is flexed, and the posterior wall sutures are tied (Figure 9-30).

The anode tube is removed, and the previously placed endotracheal tube is then advanced so that the cuff is beyond the site of the anastomosis (Figure 9-31).

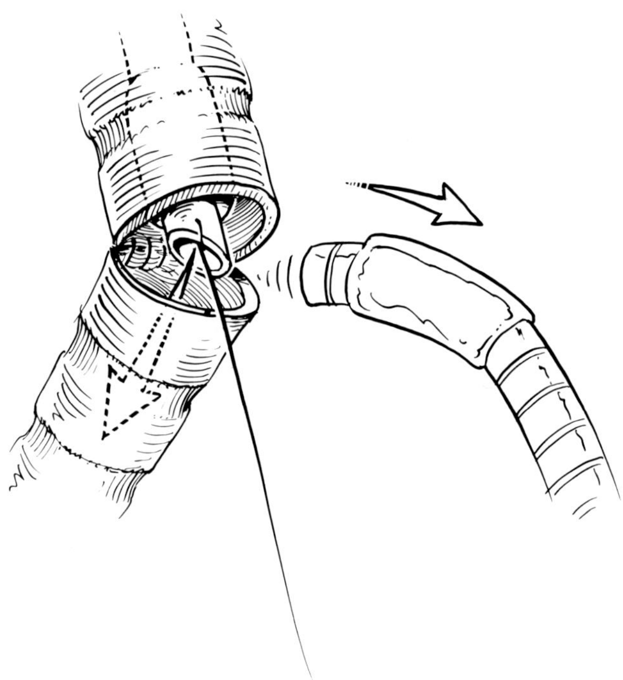

Figure 9-31

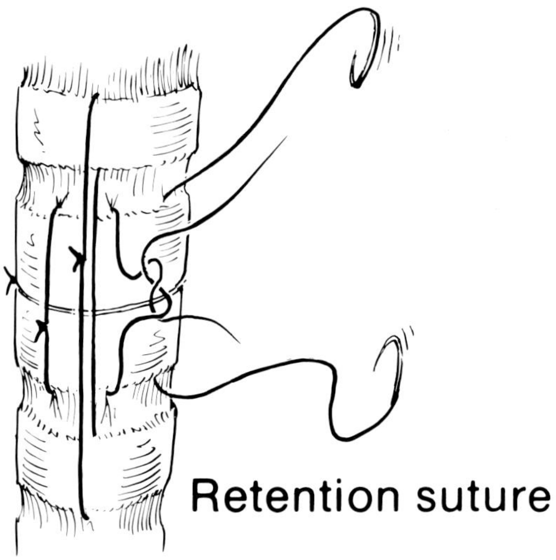

Figure 9-32

The anterior wall anastomosis is completed in a fashion similar to the posterior wall anastomosis. Retention sutures placed two rings above and below the anastomosis reduce the tension on the repair (Figure 9-32). Penrose drains are placed in the paratracheal area, the strap muscles are closed in the midline, and the skin flaps are closed in layers.

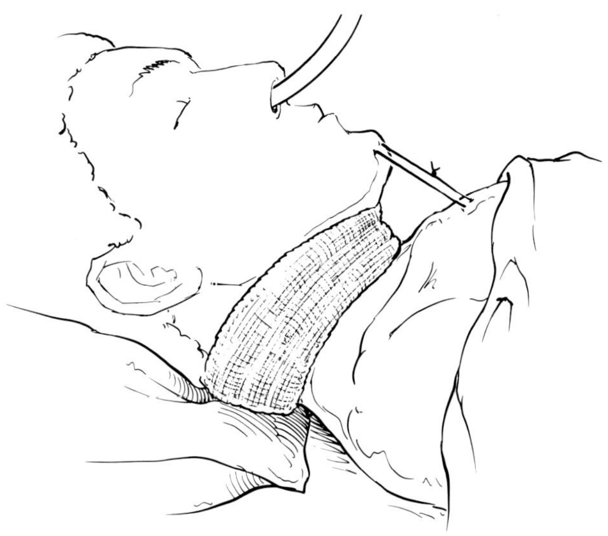

Figure 9-33

A large, nonabsorbable suture is placed through the skin and subcutaneous tissue of the chin and the presternal area in order to maintain the neck in a flexed position (Figure 9-33). The suture is left in place for 2 weeks.

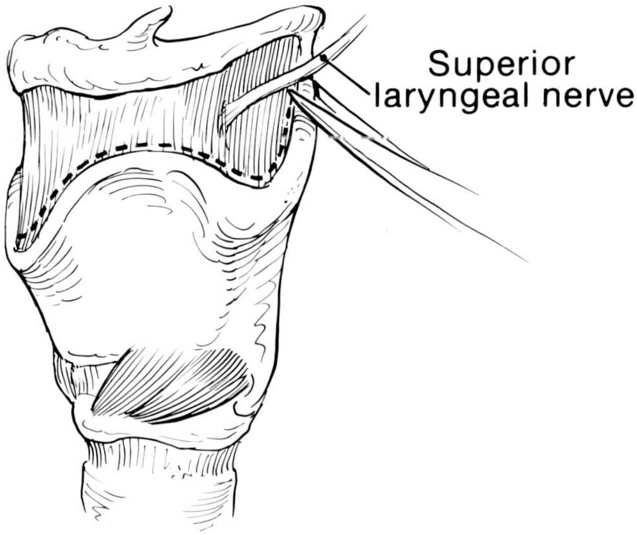

Figure 9-34

ALTERNATIVE TECHNIQUES

Another technique of laryngeal mobilization is the infrahyoid technique. An incision is made along the superior margin of the thyroid cartilage that carefully transects the thyrohyoid membrane without injuring the superior laryngeal nerves (Figure 9-34). The suspensory ligaments to the superior cornua of the thyroid cartilage are also transected.

Full mobilization of the trachea can be obtained through a thoracic approach. Techniques include division of the inferior pulmonary ligaments and reimplantation of the left mainstem bronchus into the right mainstem bronchus (Figure 9-35).

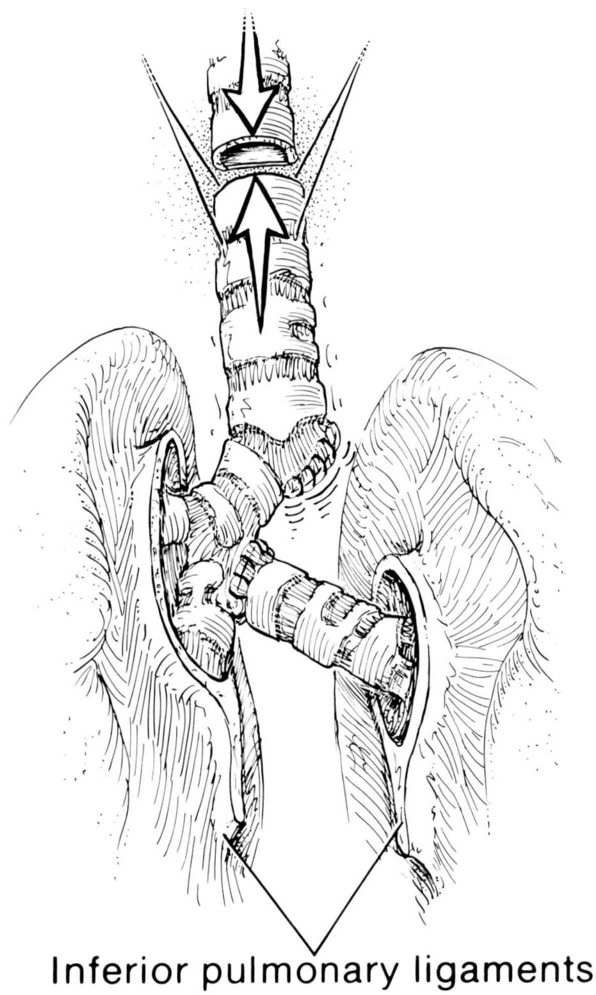

Figure 9-35

REFERENCES

1. Cohn, A. M. and Larson, D. L.: Laryngeal Injury: A Critical Review. *Arch. Otolaryngol.*, 102:166–170, 1976.
2. Dedo, H. and Fishman, N. H.: Laryngeal Release and Sleeve Resection for Tracheal Stenosis. *Ann. Otol. Rhinol. Laryngol.*, 18:285–296, 1969.
3. Grillo, H. C.: Circumferential Resection and Reconstruction of Mediastinal and Cervical Trachea. *Ann. Surg.*, 162:374–388, 1965.
4. Harris, H. H. and Tobin, H. A.: Acute Injuries of the Larynx and Trachea in 49 Patients. *Laryngoscope,* 80:1376–1384, 1970.
5. Le May, S. R.: Penetrating Wounds of the Larynx and Cervical Trachea. *Arch. Otolaryngol.*, 94:518–565, 1971.
6. Montgomery, W. W.: Suprahyoid Release for Tracheal Anastomosis. *Arch. Otolaryngol.*, 99:255–260, 1974.
7. Olson, N. R.: Surgical Treatment of Acute Blunt Laryngeal Injuries. *Ann. Otol. Rhinol. Laryngol.*, 87:716–721, 1978.
8. Sulek, M., Miller, R. H., and Mattox, K. L.: The Management of Gunshot and Stab Injuries of the Trachea. *Arch. Otolaryngol.*, 109:56–59, 1983.

Index

a
b
3 c
4 d
5 e
6 f
7 g
8 h
9 i
8 0 j